Praise for *Body Belief*

"Aimee is a beacon of hope for all looking to improve their health and awaken their best life."
— **Deepak Chopra, M.D.**

"Body Belief is must reading for every person who has ever felt sick and tired and doesn't know what's wrong. Rooted in compassion, rich with solid medical advice, and written by someone who has been there, Body Belief *is a true treasure of life-changing information that will assist anyone in healing their body and their life."*
— **Christiane Northrup, M.D.**, *New York Times* best-selling author of *Women's Bodies, Women's Wisdom*

"Aimee Raupp is one of the most kind, generous, and talented healers. Her teachings have allowed me to transform the way I think about my body and my healing path. If you are longing to reawaken your health, Body Belief *is the book you need and Aimee is the healer you want."*
— **Gabrielle Bernstein**, #1 *New York Times* best-selling author of *The Universe Has Your Back*

"Aimee's teachings are filled with an immense amount of knowledge and research combined with real-life experience and a good dose of humor. In a masterful way, she equips her clients and followers with practical tools for achieving and maintaining optimal health and vitality despite the challenges of a modern lifestyle. She pours her wisdom and expertise and infuses her clients with the healing tools of self-love and self-acceptance."
— **Agapi Stassinopoulos**, author of *Wake Up to the Joy of You*

"Aimee Raupp understands that self-love can heal all parts of you—body and soul—and she can show you the path toward whole health in all its forms."
— **Rebekah Borucki**, author of *You Have 4 Minutes to Change Your Life*

"Aimee's message is a call to action for women of all ages to take control of their health through a path of self-love. The benefits transcend physical healing, aligning body, mind, and spirit to create optimal well-being and vitality."
— **Claudia Chan**, author of *This Is How We Rise*

ALSO BY AIMEE RAUPP

Yes, You Can Get Pregnant

Chill Out & Get Healthy

Body Belief

How to Heal Autoimmune Diseases, Radically Shift Your Health, and Learn to Love Your Body More

Aimee E. Raupp,
M.S., L.Ac.

HAY HOUSE, INC.
Carlsbad, California • New York City
London • Sydney • New Delhi

Published in the United States by: Hay House, Inc.: www.hayhouse.com®
Published in Australia by: Hay House Australia Pty. Ltd.: www.hayhouse.com.au
Published in the United Kingdom by: Hay House UK, Ltd.: www.hayhouse.co.uk
Published in India by: Hay House Publishers India: www.hayhouse.co.in

Cover design: Amy Grigoriou • *Interior design:* Joe Bernier

Library of Congress has cataloged the earlier edition as follows:

Names: Raupp, Aimee E., author.
Title: Body belief : how to heal autoimmune diseases, radically shift your
    health, and learn to love your body more / Aimee E. Raupp, M.S., L.Ac.
Description: 1st edition. | Carlsbad : Hay House, Inc., 2018.
Identifiers: LCCN 2017046128 | ISBN 9781401954888 (hardback)
Subjects: LCSH: Autoimmune diseases--Psychosomatic aspects. | Women--Health
    and hygiene--Psychological aspects. | Mind and body therapies. | BISAC:
    HEALTH & FITNESS / Diseases / Immune System. | HEALTH & FITNESS /
    Women's Health. | HEALTH & FITNESS / Healthy Living.
Classification: LCC RC600 .R37 2018 | DDC 616.97/806--dc23 LC record available
at https://lccn.loc.gov/2017046128

Tradepaper ISBN: 978-1-4019-5391-1
E-book ISBN: 978-1-4019-5392-8

11 10 9 8 7 6 5 4 3
1st edition, March 2018
2nd edition, April 2019

Printed in the United States of America

To the strong women in my family who have believed in me—body, mind & soul. Your courage, grace, and guidance help me soar. Thank you~

Mommy
Nannie
Auntie
Aunt Eileen
Aunt Carolyn
Auntie Marilyn
Sister Lily
Aunt Pat
Grandma Ellen

Contents

Preface

Do you feel foggy-headed and have a hard time concentrating?

Do you wake up feeling exhausted even after sleeping eight hours?

Do your hormones feel out of whack most of the time?

Does your body ache often?

Do you regularly experience gas or bloating or indigestion?

Do you have eczema, psoriasis, or any other skin condition that will not go away?

Have you been struggling to get pregnant and/or have you had multiple miscarriages?

Do you have a hard time losing weight?

Do you go in and out of bouts of anxiety or depression?

Do you experience random environmental allergic responses, chronic sinus issues, or both?

Do you feel like you're always catching that cold that's going around the office?

If you answered "yes" to three or more of these questions and you're a woman between the ages of 20 and 45, chances are you are dealing with an autoimmune disease.

Whether you picked up this book because of an autoimmune condition you have already been diagnosed with, or you suspect you may have an autoimmune condition, or you don't feel well and want more help, you're not alone. Nearly 30 million women are dealing with an autoimmune condition like rheumatoid arthritis, Hashimoto's thyroiditis, inflammatory bowel disease, celiac sprue, endometriosis, and type 1 diabetes. And there are even more women walking around with an undiagnosed autoimmune condition, maybe even you. It is estimated that one in nine women between the ages of 20 and 45 will be diagnosed with an autoimmune disease.

Autoimmune diseases occur when the body confuses the difference between self and non-self, and attacks normal, non-sick cells by mistake and creates disease. Said another way: the body begins attacking healthy tissue because it begins to see it as unhealthy tissue, and this reaction creates inflammation and illness in the body. The American Autoimmune Related Diseases Association (AARDA) states that the incidence of autoimmune diseases have tripled over the last 40 years, affecting women—specifically women of reproductive age—at a rate 75 percent more than men. Did you catch that last part? The incidence of autoimmune diseases has tripled over the last 40 years, affecting women 75 percent more than men.

That's why I wrote this book. During my almost 15 years of clinical experience as a women's health and wellness expert, something major has become clear to me: women are suffering an autoimmune epidemic; they are walking around feeling incredibly unwell, and the problem just continues to worsen. This is not acceptable to me; nor should it be to you. That is why I developed the *Body Belief* plan—to empower you because you deserve to feel good, you are worthy of abundant health, and, most importantly, you are capable of healing yourself.

However, let me be clear: this book alone will not heal you.

This book will give you the *tools* to heal yourself, but the tools are only one part. First and foremost, this book is about you making the choice to take back your power over your health and your life. I will cheer you on along the way and give the best possible advice I have access to, but the choice to feel better has to be yours.

Are you in?

I hope you are, because in my heart of hearts I know you can and should feel better than you do right now. Together, you and I will find the path back to the thriving health of which you are worthy.

Introduction

Here's what thriving health looks like: you wake up feeling refreshed; your hormones feel balanced; you feel strong and vibrant; you digest your food well; you have a healthy, formed bowel movement every single day; your skin is hydrated with little to no blemishes (ever!), and has a refreshed glowing complexion; your hair shines; your nails grow; your body heals and recovers quickly from any setback; and most importantly, you feel nourished, stable, and supported on an emotional level.

If that's not what your health looks like now, don't fret. You can get there. I believe in your ability to radically shift your health. Even if you currently don't believe in your body and its health, I have faith in your health and your body and I will show you the way back to believing in your body again. Even if you're in the throes of dealing with some serious health issues, I can help you heal your body. I know because I have guided so many women back to optimal health. I know because I guided myself back to a state of thriving health after feeling like an ill, exhausted, puffy, hormonal mess who was itchy all over, from terrible eczema, all the time, *for years*. As a women's health and wellness expert who has been in the field of alternative medicine for 13 years, I have witnessed a lot of healing, especially when it comes to women and autoimmune diseases. In fact, I'm often the one who urges my clients to ask their Western doctors to do more tests and dig deeper, so that we can find the often-undiagnosed autoimmune condition underneath.

To be quite frank, it doesn't really matter to me what disease your Western medical doctor says you have; what matters most to me is how you feel. As a practitioner of Traditional Oriental Medicine (TOM), I use different tools than Western medical doctors do to find disease. When I diagnose a disease, I look at such things as quality of life, how well you sleep, your nutrition, your ability to manage and bounce back from stress and illness, your overall level of contentment and joy, your digestion, your energy levels, and more. And when I use the word *disease*, I am not talking about a condition that is diagnosed and treated with prescription medication. Rather, disease in my world means *dis*-ease or *dis*-comfort. Disease to me is simply a body out of sync, a body not functioning on all cylinders, a body that is moving along at below 80 percent, rather than at 95 to 100 percent. I see a lot of women who are functioning suboptimally, and since you picked up this book, chances are you're one of them.

I studied biology and chemistry in college and went on to study neuroscience in graduate school; my plans were to get a Western medical degree. I was driven to become a Western medical doctor mainly by how smart and successful it sounded in my mind. Yes, I wanted to help people—serving others was always my calling— but I also wanted the recognition and the status that came with those two letters: M.D. In hindsight, the field of Western medicine never quite suited me, and I was pushing so hard to make it work that I fell into a space of deep emotional conflict and poor health. At 19, I developed both bulimia and anorexia, all stemming from a need for perfection and not feeling adequate or secure about who I was.

My parents did what they could to help me emotionally, and were incredibly supportive, but my health struggles persisted. During my early twenties, as I continued to use my eating disorder as a coping strategy for insecurity and my deep fear of failure, I dealt with a host of health-related issues—from a raging, itchy, red, oozing skin rash that was all over my body; to daily loose bowel movements; to regular asthma and allergy flare-ups; to hormonal acne; to puffy, dark circles under my eyes; to irregular and painful periods. I felt exhausted and overwhelmed *all the time*. I was using steroid creams for my skin issues (which my doctor diagnosed as eczema), Proactiv for my acne, Pepto-Bismol regularly to soothe my constantly upset stomach, my asthma inhaler so I could breathe easily, alcohol and binge eating as a stress-management tool, and whatever other over-the-counter remedy I needed for my ailment-of-the-week.

Overall, I was in a highly dysfunctional relationship with my health. So much of it had to do with the stress I was putting myself under, all because of my hunger for the prestige of those two little letters: M.D. After a straight-talk conversation with my father, a lightbulb turned on for me. I was home from grad school for the holidays and had been out with friends for the night. I came home pretty drunk, smelling of cigarettes (back then, I had a habit of smoking a cigarette or two when I drank), and when my father greeted me at the front door he looked really disappointed in me. That night he didn't say a word, but the next day we took one of our usual father-daughter hikes and that's when he said it: "What is going on with you? You say you want to help people be healthier and live better lives, but I don't get the impression you're super healthy or happy right now. I would never go to a doctor that didn't practice what she preached."

His words really hit home. My dad and I were always the best of friends (he died in 2010 from an aggressive prostate cancer) and he knew me inside and out. With those words, he forever changed my professional and personal vision of myself. Here I was surrounded by brilliant young doctors-to-be, studying at one of the best medical institutions in the world, yet I was completely out of touch with how to doctor myself.

I began questioning everything, mainly my own approach to health. I started looking for more ways to help myself, and that's when I became a patient at the student clinic at Pacific College of Oriental Medicine (PCOM) in San Diego and was introduced to Traditional Oriental Medicine (TOM). I began taking back the power over my health—mentally and emotionally. My acupuncturist guided me to make lifestyle and dietary changes, and with her help I started on my path to healing.

My subpar health was my awakening, my red flag. Until I began feeling better, I never realized how horrible I had felt. Soon I became a patient of acupuncture and TOM, and I enrolled in PCOM's four-year master of science acupuncture program. This program, its teachings, and my dramatically improved health forever shifted the way I view medicine and doctoring. Through the acupuncture program's mandatory first-year psychology track, where the focus is healing yourself before healing anyone else, I finally overcame my eating disorders.

Now, almost 20 years after my health reawakening, I am prepared to guide you back to optimal health. But before we dive into the *Body Belief* way, let's first talk about something that's very important to me and is the through-line of my professional practice and my life: self-love. I know it's a cliché these days to talk about self-love, but it was the cornerstone of my transformation, and in order for you to make your own meaningful health shifts, it needs to be the cornerstone of yours.

When I am talking about self-love, what I really mean is being kind, gentle, and compassionate toward yourself. Self-love is patience; it is understanding; it is forgiveness. Loving yourself takes you from a place of harsh self-judgment to a place of allowing yourself to be imperfect and of being open to receiving the guidance you deserve. And here is the first gift of self-love: don't kill yourself if you don't do it perfectly right away, all of the time, every second of every minute. Do the best you can do right now, and strive to do better each day. If you follow my recommendations even just 70 to 80 percent of the time, you will still see results. Of course, the more committed you are, the faster you will see your health shift and the more lasting your transformation will be. But through all of this, be easy on yourself. Accept right now that there will be ebbs and flows, and moments where your health isn't thriving the way you want. There will be times when you're not as committed to this plan as you want to be. And that's OK. We are all human, and I am not talking about striving for perfection. I am talking about finding balance in your life, so that you can feel better than you do now.

Take me, *the health expert,* for example. There are times when I don't follow my dietary recommendations, or when I fall out of my regular meditation habit, or when I let stress get the best of me, or when I am working longer hours and getting less sleep. The difference between now and back when I was in really poor health is that now I can feel it immediately when my body is in *dis*-ease or *dis*-comfort, through what I call my red flags. Red flags are problematic or uncomfortable symptoms that you are dealing with on a fairly regular basis. One of my major red-flag symptoms is eczema—a red, itchy skin rash that no topical cream of any kind really helps. When my eczema begins to flare up, it's a clear-cut sign that I am not connected to my body and the health routines that support it. In fact, not that long ago I had a flare-up of my eczema, and it was a great lesson for me.

Recently I gave birth to my first child. It's truly been one of the most amazing times in my life, as I am just so blissed-out and so in love with my baby, my husband, and my life. But I began pushing myself to health-compromising limits: breastfeeding and pumping, working full time, running my business and my three clinics, working on this book, striving for (unattainable) perfection in the work-life department, moving out of New York City, and being present and on for my husband, my clients, my family, my friends, and myself.

I set out on a mission to make the eczema go away. My diet had been stellar while I was breastfeeding, but I tweaked it even more. I tried taking extra supplements. I went to my acupuncturist and began taking an herbal formula. I started meditating more. But nothing really worked.

I honestly couldn't figure it out until the eczema appeared with a vengeance on my right breast. At that time my son had been exclusively breastfed for a solid seven months, and as we were heading into month eight, I was considering cutting back some and introducing formula. But the truth was I felt guilty about it. Really, really guilty. I felt as if I would be judged by others for my decision to cut back on breastfeeding. I was comparing myself to other women who breastfed exclusively for 12 months or longer. It felt like if I were to add formula, I was taking from my child to give to myself. The little voice in my head was telling me I was being selfish, and that didn't feel good at all. Through my meditation, I heard my father's voice telling me I wasn't completely practicing what I preach, as I was keeping in all of my emotions. I wasn't sharing my feelings of guilt and shame with anyone. Then one day, not long after that meditation, a dear friend pried, asking me, *the health expert*, why I thought my skin was flaring up. Through sudden, uncontrollable tears, I blurted out, "I think I need to stop breastfeeding, but I feel incredibly guilty about it!"

In that moment I found the reason for my red-flag flare-up.

It wasn't until I worked through my self-judgment that my eczema began to subside. Now I can see that I was putting too much pressure on myself to "do it all," and that that was the root of my rashy-skin flare-up. My red flag (literally my red-rash–flag) flare-up wasn't caused by the usual things that affect me, such as too much sugar, sleep deprivation, or skipping my meditation or my exercise; it was guilt, and being disconnected from who I was in that moment: a woman who wanted to stop breastfeeding at eight months. I was not practicing self-love or kindness. I was not being forgiving toward myself. Rather, I was harshly judging and attacking myself for my decision. Even though I am always the one who tells others to do the best they can, I knew I was being very, very critical of myself.

Do you know what it feels like to be disconnected from yourself? It's that feeling that you're keeping a secret, like you're shying away from what you really want to do or say.

I know some of you are dealing with health issues that are way more intense than the eczema flare-up I had on my breast. But, at the core, I can confidently say that whenever our health issues come up, whatever they are, we have a few things in common: we are disconnected from our bodies, we are believing unkind things about ourselves and our bodies, and we are exposing our bodies to too many toxins, both emotional and physical.

In order to heal and thrive, we all must

1. RECONNECT to our bodies spiritually, emotionally and physically

2. RENEW our beliefs about our body and our health

3. REAWAKEN our health through eliminating environmental toxins (remember, environmental toxins are not just chemicals or pesticides— they include emotional toxins too, such as toxic relationships)

Let me break these down for you so you are clear on what I'm talking about:

When we are disconnected from our bodies, there is a loss of communication to the physical, emotional, and spiritual aspects of who we are. At the very root of autoimmunity is the body's not recognizing itself, and therefore mistakenly attacking itself. This inability to distinguish self from non-self isn't purely a physical or cellular issue; it is an emotional and spiritual one.

The first and most significant pillar of the *Body Belief* plan is to RECONNECT to yourself. When you reconnect and reestablish a kinder, more compassionate relationship with yourself, you can then tune into any skewed beliefs or thought patterns you have formed about your body and your health. One of the big takeaways I want you to receive from this book is that your beliefs dictate your behavior, and your behavior dictates your health. Shifting the conversation you have with yourself in the privacy of your own mind, and thereby renewing your deep-rooted body beliefs, will allow your behaviors to shift and your health to thrive. Why? Because your body hears everything your brain says.

The second pillar of this book is to RENEW your body beliefs, because we all have formed beliefs about our bodies and our health that we have accepted as truths. Moreover, we tell these beliefs to the trillions of cells in our bodies thousands of times each day. Some of the beliefs we have the habit of telling to our body and all the cells that inhabit it are things like: "I'm old and that's why my body is failing me." Or, "My mom was sick and that's why I'm sick. It's genetic." Or, "What can I expect, I don't treat my body well so I feel like crap because of it." Or, "I'm always sick. That's never going to change." Or, "The doctor told me there's no cure. There's nothing I can do." Such beliefs about your body don't serve you, and they definitely don't allow you to heal. You are worthy of feeling better, but in order to do so, you must first change that conversation you are having about your body and its health. Current neuroscience research shows that your beliefs dictate your behavior and your behavior dictates your health.[1]

Body Belief will show you how to renew your beliefs about your body and its health, because if you believe that feeling subpar is good enough, then you are going to make lifestyle choices that support feeling subpar. And guess what? You deserve to feel better than subpar.

The third pillar of the *Body Belief* plan is to REAWAKEN your health by shifting your lifestyle to eradicate your exposure to environmental toxins on every level: emotional, physical, and nutritional. The Western medical research is clear: environmental chemicals and stressors are linked to the prevalence of autoimmune disease. I will discuss potential environmental toxins from pesticides in food; to noxious substances in home, bath, and beauty products; to workplace stressors; to poor sleeping habits; to toxic thoughts and emotions—and show you how to adjust your lifestyle so you can improve your health fast.

I've got your back. I will coach you every step of the way. You are ready to take ownership of a new health-transforming belief:

*"I have the power to change my beliefs
and radically shift my health."*

When we are connected to ourselves and believe in our bodies and our health, we treat our body like the temple that it is. You may be dealing with less than optimal health or living in a state of dis-ease, but that doesn't have to devastate your life. Your dis-ease does not have to define you. Through reconnecting to yourself and renewing your beliefs about your body, you can reawaken your health and triumph over your illness. You have the power to radically shift your health, and the *Body Belief* plan will enable you to do it.

Chapter One

Autoimmunity: A Hostile Takeover of Your Body

Autoimmune disease is a case of misidentification. It's basically an identity crisis at the cellular level, the manifestation of cellular hostility outweighing cellular kindness. Sure, there are a lot of moving parts and a ton of cellular cues that need to happen before your body shows signs of autoimmunity, but in very simple laymen's terms, it's a hostile takeover. One that is affecting you and millions of other women.

The American Autoimmune Related Diseases Association (AARDA) estimates that 30 million American women have at least one diagnosed autoimmune disease. Worse, many women are walking around feeling unwell and are completely unaware that they may have an autoimmune disease. For example, it is estimated that only 5 percent of those who suffer with celiac disease (one of the most common autoimmune diseases) have actually been diagnosed with it[1]—meaning there are scores of people walking around with an inability to digest gluten and they don't even know it. The why's and the how's of autoimmune diseases are still a bit of a mystery to the Western medical community.

Because there are more than 100 confirmed autoimmune conditions presenting as a collection of vague symptoms, many medical practitioners misdiagnose them or don't diagnose them at all. A typical scenario for millions of women goes like this: you feel exhausted, your body hurts in places it never did before, you have dark circles under your eyes, your hormones seem all out of whack, and it only continues to get worse. You visit your doctor and they do some blood work, where everything comes back within normal parameters. Your doctor tells you there is nothing wrong with you. You drag on, moving through your days feeling even more exhausted; your whole body aches and your head feels like it's in a fog. You see another doctor, and it's the same thing: blood work appears normal and you are told there is nothing wrong with you. Next you see a specialist, and it's the same thing: all labs tests are normal, and even though you feel exhausted and depressed, have daily headaches, and suffer pain all through your body, your doctor will tell you there is nothing wrong and perhaps you're just overworked or underslept, or "It's all in your head."

The average autoimmune patient sees six different doctors over an average of five years before receiving a diagnosis. Moreover, 45 percent of patients with serious autoimmune conditions such as celiac disease, scleroderma, lupus, Hashimoto's thyroiditis, and Crohn's disease have a very difficult time getting a diagnosis and instead are labeled as hypochondriacs by their doctors (in the chart notes, not to their face).[2]

But it doesn't stop there. Once you do finally get a diagnosis, there are not many treatment options from a Western medical perspective that can help you. The ones available involve steroids and immunosuppressants, which have their own host of side effects and are incredibly punishing to the body.

The incidence of autoimmune illnesses continues to rise. Since the 1980s it has tripled, and affects women 75 percent more than it does men. You may have picked up this book because you have already been diagnosed with an autoimmune condition, suspect you may have one, or just really want to feel better regardless of your diagnosis. The *Body Belief* plan will transform your health and allow your body not only to heal but to thrive. But before I get into how, let's talk more about what autoimmunity is, so you can have a better understanding of what your body is going through.

What Is Autoimmunity?

From a Western scientific standpoint, autoimmunity occurs when your body's immune system begins attacking normal, healthy tissue. Your body's immune system exists to destroy foreign invaders; it is there to protect your body from bad bacteria, viruses, and any other potentially harmful pathogens that are not supposed to be in your body. It's imperative to your survival to have a properly functioning immune system, since your body is exposed to potential invaders all the time. But in a body with autoimmunity, your immune system begins to attack and destroy the same tissues it's meant to protect.

Any number of things can go awry, and when they do, your immune system can no longer differentiate you (self) from invader (non-self) and starts assaulting every cell and protein in your body indiscriminately. This flurry of assaults results in chronic inflammation and eventually an autoimmune disease.

In autoimmunity, your immune system is working perfectly fine; the problem is more that parts of your immune system have been targeted to attack specific parts of the body in the same manner they would be targeted to attack a foreign invader. Your immune system is doing what it's supposed to do, but it has been triggered to target proteins and cells that were once considered safe. This miscommunication leads to whole-body inflammation. This triggers autoimmunity, which in turn causes other physical symptoms.

If you want more information on how your immune system works, and the exact details on how an autoimmune disease arises in your body, I recommend you read The Paleo Approach: Reverse Autoimmune Disease and Heal Your Body *by Sarah Ballantyne, Ph.D. (New York: Victory Belt Publishing, 2013). Dr. Ballantyne is a medical biophysicist who has studied autoimmunity extensively, and her teachings are not only innovative but realistic from a Western medical perspective.*

What is inflammation?

First off, inflammation isn't always a bad thing. Think about when you get a splinter. If you leave the splinter in, the area where it is gets red, swollen, and painful, and it usually feels hot to the touch. The reason this reaction takes place is that when the splinter entered your finger, your body was alerted that there was a foreign invader, so it sent out a host of immune system cells to kill the infection. The concentration of these immune cells in the area of the splinter created the red, swollen, and painful finger. If you didn't go in and physically remove the splinter, these cells would remain and create a barrier between the splinter and the rest of your body as a means of self-preservation. This type of acute inflammation is a result of your body's immune system effectively doing its job of protecting your body from foreign invaders.

We want our bodies to attack foreign invaders so we can fight off colds, viruses, injuries, allergic reactions, and any other pesky environmental invaders. Inflammation in these acute situations facilitates healing, but it gets troublesome when it's chronic, as in the case when the body is constantly under attack from foreign invaders, psychological stress, lack of sleep, poor diet, and/or environmental toxins. Chronic inflammation is at the root of autoimmune diseases, and ridding the body of this inflammation is what the *Body Belief* plan is all about.

The reasons for the miscommunication are layered. Western medicine usually attributes autoimmune conditions to:

1. Genetics

2. Past infections

3. Environmental toxins

So even though you may have a genetic predisposition to getting an autoimmune illness, depending on how you live your life and other epigenetic factors, the disease will or will not affect you because your genes are not set in stone. Alternatively, you might have had a previous infection like H. pylori or Epstein-Barr virus, and that infection coupled with how you live your life and other environmental influences could trigger the miscommunication, resulting in an autoimmune condition.

Let's break these three reasons down further so you can really get a handle on what's going on.

The genetic part you can't change. But as we now know because of the science of epigenetics, you can influence how your genes express themselves by making different lifestyle changes. I will discuss epigenetics more in Chapter 2, but know this: how you live your life and the environmental toxins you are exposed to can determine whether or not certain genes turn on and you get a disease you're genetically predisposed to. When it comes to your genetics, keep in mind that "fewer than 10% of those individuals with an increased genetic susceptibility (of autoimmune diseases) actually develop clinical disease. This suggests a strong environmental trigger in the pre-autoimmune process. Environmental factors are also likely to affect the outcome of the process and the rate of progression to disease in those individuals who develop autoimmunity."[3]

Your history of infections, similarly to your genetics, can't be undone. But as Sarah Ballantyne, Ph.D., states in her book *The Paleo Approach*, "It's important to understand the distinction between infection contributing to the development of autoimmune disease and causing it . . . Autoimmune diseases are not caused by infectious organisms. Instead, infections increase your chances of developing specific autoimmune diseases."[4]

And then there are the environmental toxins. Fred Miller, director of the Environmental Autoimmunity Group at the National Institute of Environmental Health Sciences, states that autoimmune diseases are now recognized as among the leading causes of death among young and middle-aged women in the United States. He insists that the reasons are largely environmental, meaning that our lifestyle and diet are the root cause of autoimmunity. In an article published in the journal *Environmental Health Perspectives*, Miller claims, "Our gene sequences aren't changing fast enough to account for the increases [of autoimmune diseases]. Yet our environment is—we've got 80,000 chemicals approved for use in commerce, but we know very little about their immune effects. Our lifestyles are also different than they were a few decades ago, and we're eating more processed food."[5] Virginia T. Ladd, president and executive director of AARDA, states, "With the rapid increase in autoimmune diseases, it clearly suggests that environmental factors are at play . . . Genes do not change in such a short period of time."[6]

A review of the topic of autoimmunity in the journal *Environmental Health Perspectives* states that scientists define environmental triggers broadly, but chemicals, infectious agents, stress, hormones, drugs, diet, weight gain, behavior, and more have all been cited as etiological factors leading to the increasing incidence of autoimmune diseases and their diagnosis.

These autoimmune-provoking toxins include toxic foods, toxic thoughts, toxic relationships, toxic skincare routines, toxic prescription medications, and toxic chemicals in the air you breathe. From my many years of clinical experience, I have found that there are three main ways that environmental toxins affect your health and cause autoimmunity: your brain and your beliefs about your health, the food you eat, and how you interact in your world. Let's break these down.

Your Brain, Beliefs, and Autoimmunity

The conversation you have with yourself in the privacy of your own mind affects your health at the cellular level. Why? Because your brain hears everything you say to your body. As there are 37 trillion cells in your body, the question becomes: Are you cheering them on with loving thoughts, or verbally abusing them with toxic thoughts? If the root of autoimmunity is your body attacking itself on a cellular level, are you attacking yourself with toxic thoughts on an emotional level?

Your thoughts create chemical messengers in your brain, and your body responds to them.[7] If you think, "I am happy," a chemical messenger then conveys that to your body and all of your trillions of cells. The same thing happens if you think "I am stressed out" or "I am so unhappy" or "I hate my body." It also happens if you are thinking things like, "I hate my job" or "I am always sick" or "My body never does what I want it to do."

Contemplate the following from stem-cell biologist and author of *The Biology of Belief* Bruce Lipton:

> The cells [in your body] are maintained by a culture medium, popularly known as blood. The brain is the regulatory organ that regulates and maintains the chemical composition of the blood. The brain's control of the blood's chemistry is linked to our perceptions (mind) and emotions (reflecting chemical signals in the blood). When you have a perception of love, the brain releases oxytocin (love hormone that regulates body's metabolism and supports growth), serotonin and growth hormone, ALL chemicals that when added to cells in a culture dish will enhance growth and health of the cells. In contrast, when a person is in fear, their brain releases stress hormones (cortisol, norepinephrine and histamine) that shut down a cell's growth processes and inhibits the immune system, which happens to be completely unsustainable for life.[8]

The average person has about fifty thousand thoughts each day, and each thought influences the chemical messengers in your brain and how your body functions. That means your thoughts are a part of your illness *and* your wellness. The *Body Belief* plan will reconnect you to yourself and renew your body beliefs so that you can begin to hear the conversation you are having with yourself, change the tone of it from one of hostility to one of kindness, and create a loving environment in your body for your health to thrive.

Your Food and Autoimmunity

Seventy percent of your immune system is in the tissues surrounding your gastrointestinal (GI) tract,[9] since it regularly interacts with the external environment through the foods you eat, the beverages you drink, and anything else you put in your mouth. A large part of your immune system is in your stomach, small intestine, and large intestine. Autoimmune research shows that "the loss of the protective function of the mucosal barriers that interact with the environment (mainly the gastrointestinal lining) is necessary for autoimmunity to develop. . . The autoimmune process can be arrested if the interplay between genes and environmental triggers is prevented by re-establishing intestinal barrier function."[10] What this means is that the lining of the GI tract is compromised in an autoimmune disease, and in order to heal it must be fixed through dietary changes.

This condition is called increased intestinal permeability, also known as leaky gut. Just as your skin is a barrier to the outside world, the lining of your intestines is a barrier within your body to the outside world. In a perfectly healthy body, what you eat goes into your intestinal tract and is broken down into useable components by dozens of enzymes, acids, and friendly bacteria that live in your gut. Once most of the food is broken down, it is moved by certain cells from inside your intestinal tract to areas throughout your body, so that your body can receive nutrition. The food that's not broken down into its simplest components gets excreted as waste in the form of poop and pee. In a body with autoimmunity, the science shows that the intestinal barrier gets leaky, so food particles and other substances that were in your food, like bacteria or toxic pesticides, that normally would be excreted as waste actually get absorbed into your body.[11]

A leaky gut has been present in every autoimmune condition that has been tested.[12] Certain foods in your diet—particularly ones like glutinous grains (wheat, barley, and rye), beans (yes, every kind of bean), and nightshade vegetables (white potatoes, peppers, tomatoes, and eggplant)—seem to cause the gastrointestinal lining to become leaky.[13] The *Body Belief* plan is going to give you exactly what you need to know about what foods to eat and not to eat so you can heal your gut and your autoimmunity.

Your World and Autoimmunity

Autoimmune diseases as a whole are considered a modern disease because their incidence is steadily increasing *only* in modernized nations. You see, the world you live in and how you interact with that world affects your health and ultimately your autoimmunity. It seems all the luxuries of the modern world—including the skincare products you use, the relationships you keep, the air you breathe, how much you sleep, how you manage your stress, how much you work, your exercise routine, and what you are believing about your body and its wellness (or illness)—all have a major effect on your health and the manifestation of autoimmunity. What autoimmune research scientists are seeing is that the environmental toxins provide the most clear-cut correlation with the incidence and rise of autoimmune conditions.[14] That is why the *Body Belief* plan is going to teach you straightforward ways to reduce your exposure to such toxins. You will be provided with tips and tools to better understand how your interaction with your world is influencing your health and how to shift toward more optimal health and healing.

The Red-Flag Symptoms of Autoimmune Diseases

Take a moment to go through these symptoms and honestly check off all of the ones you are currently feeling. After following the *Body Belief* program for at least eight weeks, I want you to come back to this list and see how many of your red flags have lessened or gone away entirely. Use the symptoms on this list as a tracker of your healing progress. As you see these symptoms begin to shift, you will know that your body is responding to the *Body Belief* plan and healing is underway!

Please keep in mind: not all of these symptoms individually indicate an autoimmune condition; it's when three or more of these symptoms occur for you on a regular basis (three or more times a week) that they are indicators of chronic inflammation, which can lead to an autoimmune condition.

THE GOAL: Follow the *Body Belief* plan for at least eight weeks (ideally, forever!) and see your red flags begin to lessen and disappear. Keep revisiting this list to remind yourself of all the changes that are happening in your body by following the *Body Belief* plan!

- [ ] Headaches
- [ ] Anxiety
- [ ] Depression
- [ ] Nervousness
- [ ] Irritability
- [ ] Brain fog
- [ ] Dizziness
- [ ] Memory problems
- [ ] Mood swings
- [ ] Slurred or stuttered speech
- [ ] Attention-deficit problems
- [ ] Body rashes, red bumps on facial skin, and/or red flaking skin
- [ ] Thick red patches, covered with scales, on your skin
- [ ] Skin that looks shiny on the hands and forearms
- [ ] Acne
- [ ] Hives
- [ ] Rosacea
- [ ] Eczema
- [ ] Psoriasis
- [ ] Dermatitis
- [ ] Dry, scaly skin
- [ ] Yellowing on the skin and/or whites of the eyes
- [ ] Allergies
- [ ] Chest congestion
- [ ] Shortness of breath
- [ ] Difficulty breathing
- [ ] Asthma
- [ ] Dry mouth
- [ ] Excessive thirst

- [ ] Chronic cough
- [ ] Frequent throat clearing
- [ ] Sore throat
- [ ] Swollen lips
- [ ] Frequent colds
- [ ] Thyroid issues (previously diagnosed)
- [ ] Anemia
- [ ] Fatigue
- [ ] Hyperactivity
- [ ] Heart palpitations
- [ ] Feeling faint
- [ ] Easy weight gain
- [ ] Excessive hunger
- [ ] Sudden and/or easy weight loss
- [ ] No appetite
- [ ] Compulsive eating
- [ ] Food cravings
- [ ] Water retention/swelling in ankles
- [ ] General feeling of malaise and/or weakness
- [ ] Cold hands and feet
- [ ] Fingers and toes that turn red, white, or blue in response to heat or cold
- [ ] Easy sweating
- [ ] Hot flashes
- [ ] Brittle hair
- [ ] Brittle nails
- [ ] Slow-healing sores
- [ ] Easy bruising
- [ ] Mouth sores
- [ ] Muscle pain and weakness
- [ ] Joint pain
- [ ] Red, hot, swollen joints
- [ ] Stiff, swollen, and/or deformed joints

- [ ] Trouble with balance and coordination
- [ ] Stiffness and pain in your muscles
- [ ] Feeling "wired and tired"
- [ ] Blurry vision or seeing floaters in your eyes
- [ ] Swollen eyes
- [ ] Dark circles under eyes
- [ ] Watery, itchy eyes
- [ ] Nasal congestions
- [ ] Excessive nasal mucus
- [ ] Stuffy/runny nose
- [ ] Frequent sneezing
- [ ] Itchy ears
- [ ] Ear infections
- [ ] Ringing in ears
- [ ] Hearing loss
- [ ] Exhaustion
- [ ] Insomnia or trouble sleeping
- [ ] Stomach cramping or pain
- [ ] Nausea/vomiting
- [ ] Heartburn
- [ ] Gas
- [ ] Bloated stomach
- [ ] Diarrhea
- [ ] Constipation
- [ ] Rectal bleeding
- [ ] Missed or irregular menstrual periods
- [ ] Fertility challenges and/ or miscarriages
- [ ] Frequent colds
- [ ] Frequent or urgent urination
- [ ] Genital itchiness
- [ ] Anal itchiness
- [ ] Genital discharge

TOM and Autoimmunity

One last thing before we begin the *Body Belief* plan: I want to explain to you how I was trained to view autoimmune conditions from a Traditional Oriental Medicine (TOM) perspective. In TOM, we don't focus on what a Western medical diagnosis would focus on. Rather, we focus on how the patient feels and their symptoms. When I work with clients, I do a complete health history intake covering everything from how you sleep to how you poop to what you eat and what supplements you take to how you feel emotionally. TOM is a completely holistic approach to health. We see the body and mind as one, and with that every single dis-ease manifestation takes that into account. There is no separation of physical and emotional. In TOM, there is also no such thing as the immune system existing separately from the body and mind as a whole.

When it comes to working with autoimmune conditions, I rely solely on how the patient presents to me from a TOM perspective, what red-flag symptoms they have, and how I can get to the root of the problem so healing can happen. The way I was taught to approach any illness was to find the root cause of the dis-ease and treat from that place. Whereas the Western medical model mainly treats the symptoms, or what TOM calls *branches*, TOM treats the root of the problem.

For instance, whereas Western medicine will give you an antacid to treat heartburn, TOM will address the mental, emotional, physical, and nutritional aspects of the dis-ease and work to restore the proper digestive functioning so that the heartburn goes away on its own. When it comes to autoimmune illnesses, there are many facets of the body—mental, emotional, physical, and nutritional—that can experience dis-ease or discomfort. Accordingly, I am not just treating the aching pain in your knee or your sleep issues or your constipation; I am digging deep to get to the root of why all of these dis-eases and discomforts have arisen, as they are not separate: they came from the same root disturbance in your body.

From a TOM perspective, there are three very important vital substances that everyone has and that, taken together, we see as the cornerstone of health and vitality. Rectifying them is the key to healing *any* dis-ease:

1. Qi

2. Blood

3. Essence

Qi (pronounced "chi") is what TOM considers to be the vital force or energy that drives life. The Chinese symbol for qi depicts it as the steam that rises above rice as you cook it. Qi is like a warm mist that circulates through the body, giving it life; it is found in any living thing. Qi is derived from two main sources: the air we breathe and the food we eat. In TOM, qi is believed to flow through the body via channels, or *meridians*, that correspond to particular organs or organ systems. When qi becomes imbalanced or blocked, then dis-eases can arise. In TOM we say that all pain or discomfort is a sign that qi is blocked, and that acupuncture works by unblocking stuck qi. The blockage of qi can also inhibit the functioning of any organ in the body, also resulting in illness. The secret to thriving health is to generate abundant qi by means of a nutritious diet, clean air, and the unimpeded circulation of qi.

The second most important substance crucial to sustaining health and vitality in TOM is blood. Where qi is more of a warm mist that fills up the body, blood is a liquid that moves through the vessels of the body. Blood is the foundational element for the formation of bones, nerves, skin, muscles, and organs. It nourishes the body, moistens body tissues, and ensures that they do not dry out. Blood also has an effect on the mental/emotional facet of the body as it is said to contain the spirit. From a TOM viewpoint, when a person is lacking blood, their body shows symptoms of deficiency and they often feel fatigued and a lack of spirit or liveliness.

The third most important vital substance in TOM is essence or *Jing*, the substance responsible for reproduction and regeneration. It derives from two sources: the energy inherited from one's parents (similar to the genetics in Western medicine) and the energy a person acquires in his or her daily life (chiefly from air, food, and water). Jing regulates the body's growth and development, and works with qi to help protect the body from harmful external factors.

When it comes to the treatment of autoimmunity, all three of these vital substances come into play. One of my teachers, Subhuti Dharmananda, describes it thus: "If the vessels were full of qi and blood, and the organs working properly and full of their essences, the person would be healthy, or might, at the worst, suffer minor and short-term diseases. Instead, the [longstanding] deficiency [of qi, blood, and essence] allows external pathogenic influences to enter, and permits the [autoimmune] disease to progress, transform, and become serious because of inadequate resistance to this process by [healthy, abundant] qi.[15]

What this means in modern-day layman's terms is that all three vital substances are compromised in a person who shows signs of an autoimmune condition. When qi, blood, and essence are deficient, the body becomes much more susceptible to the influence of the environment and its toxins. In TOM we see the biggest assaults on qi, blood, and essence as coming from overexertion, overwork, too much alcohol, smoking, recreational drugs, prescription drugs, excessive sexual activity, loud music, violent movies, repressed emotions, a lack of peace in one's life, processed foods, lack of sleep, and a disconnect from nature. Therefore, healing autoimmunity from a TOM perspective is all about adopting a nutrient-dense diet and regulating lifestyle and emotions to emphasize peace, calm, and self-appreciation in one's life. And that is exactly what the Body Belief plan is going to direct you to do.

Now that you have a clearer understanding of what it means to have an autoimmune condition, I want you to take a moment and speak to your body in a loving, kind way, and remind it of something very important: you have the power to change your health and heal from autoimmunity.

There are many layers to what your body is going through, and we are going to analyze and work through each of them. Let's do this because you are worth it!

Chapter Two

○

Belief Is Key

I know you picked up this book because you want to feel better. And now you know that a key to optimizing your health is a belief in your body and its ability to heal. So, tell me:

Do you believe you are capable of feeling better?
Do you believe your health can thrive?
Do you believe your body can heal?

I have written *Body Belief* because I believe in you. I believe in your body. I believe the teachings I offer can radically transform your health. But none of that matters if you don't believe your health can be radically transformed.

What do you believe about your health and your body's capacity for healing? Perhaps you believe that you can and will feel better, or maybe you believe there is no hope for you. Maybe you take your health for what it is, accepting it rather than challenging it or questioning your beliefs. Maybe you have never even been asked, or have never asked yourself, about your health beliefs. We all have beliefs about our health whether we know it or not, and we are making choices every day based upon those beliefs. In this chapter I am going to help you get to the core of what you believe about your health, so that you can make lasting changes. I am here to help you unveil your health beliefs, because until you do, this book—*in fact, any book*—can't offer you the healing you are longing for.

First off, let's discuss what a belief is. Famed 19th-century Russian author and playwright Anton Chekhov said, "Man is what he believes."

So, simply stated, a belief is a thought you judge to be true. Beliefs are the mental architecture of how you move through the world; they form your guiding principles and judgments about how the world works, how you work, your place in the world, and how you interact with the world. The beliefs, judgments, and thoughts you believe to be true can propel you forward or hold you back. Let's break down the three main ways your beliefs do this.

1) Your Beliefs Dictate Your Behavior, and Your Behavior Dictates Your Health

Your underlying and mostly unconscious beliefs dictate your daily thoughts and actions. How? Perhaps as a child you witnessed your mom become ill and your mother's illness led directly to your belief that all mothers are ill, or all women are sick, and as you grew into womanhood you believed that that must be your lot in life, so you don't bother to honor your health by sleeping enough or exercising because you don't believe it will make any difference. And you befriend other sick women, because that is your model of what women are. Or, if you supported your best friend as she beat breast cancer, you believe breast cancer is beatable, and you make sure to eat lots of green vegetables, take antioxidant supplements, see your doctors regularly for checkups, are first in line at breast cancer walks, and proudly share your friend's story with anyone you can. Or you were raised by someone who overate when they were stressed out, and the connection was made for you then that overeating is the way you should handle stress, so now you do the same thing; you even found a romantic partner who does the same thing and you handle stress that way together. Or you watched your father go to work every day to a job he hated and then come home exhausted and demoralized, complaining about how working hard gets you nowhere in life, so as an adult you have now fallen into that same pattern: tired, stressed, and bitter about your work life.

I bet one of these examples resonated with you. It's exactly how what you believe about your health impacts your health, your behaviors around your health, how you interact in your world, and your ability to change your health, heal, and thrive.

If you're like most people, you're not consciously aware of your repetitive thoughts and beliefs. Most of you don't even realize how often you say your health beliefs and personal philosophies out loud in casual settings (think social gatherings, dinner parties, girls' nights, break rooms at work, or mommy groups). Have you heard yourself saying anything like, "I'm always sick," "I'm going to get diabetes, everyone in my family gets it," "Cancer runs in my family; it's inevitable," "My dad gave me his gene for heart attacks," "I have my mother's knees; I'll need a replacement soon." Whatever it is, I am sure you have some type of ingrained beliefs about your health. I'm sure you think them *and* outwardly share them with others, a lot. Know that they are shifting your life and your health, because these beliefs are affecting your brain, your body, and your daily behaviors. We talked about this above and in the last chapter, but I want to reiterate it because it's that important: you think about fifty thousand thoughts each day that influence the chemical messengers in your brain, how your body functions, and the life choices you make. Your thoughts are a part of your illness *and* your wellness. I want you to start owning that truth.

2) Your Beliefs Affect the Chemicals in Your Brain and How Your Body Functions

Plain and simple: your beliefs affect the functioning of the trillions of cells in your body. Yes, really! Take that in. I already touched upon this in the last chapter, but as I know it's a new way of seeing things, I'll go over it again. Your thoughts trigger chemical messengers in your brain, which in turn trigger your cells to take action. To really understand how this works, we are going to revisit a concept that we all learned in high school science class: the "fight-or-flight" response. This response is something all animals have, and it is triggered when an animal is faced with a predator, one that may kill or eat it. In this situation, the animal has two choices: to fight the predator or to run away. The animal's body is flooded with hormones to give it the ability to do one or the other.

We human animals have that same response, and it is triggered every day of our life. Let's say you really messed up at work, like made a really huge mistake. You know you need to tell your boss, and then suddenly you see your boss approaching from down the hall, and your boss looks mad. You think, "OK, I could run away or confront that big scary boss." Your heart rate elevates, you may start to sweat, stress hormones in your body kick in, and then you react either by running back to your desk (flight) or standing your ground and confronting your boss (fight). And this was all triggered just by your seeing your boss and thinking a thought.

You don't need to be in a near-death situation for this response to be set off; you need only to be thinking a stressful thought like, "Oh crap, I screwed up at work and I have to deal with it," or, "The bills keep rolling in and I don't have enough money in my checking account," or, "I have zero energy to get through the day, how can I even think about managing my career and my family," or, "I can't tolerate going to visit my family because they are just going to ask me, again, what is going on in my life." You get it.

A stressful thought, a belief, creates a chemical cascade in your brain that then triggers the release of hormones in your body, causing your body and its cells to experience fear—to think it's under attack—and it has to either flee the situation or fight back *immediately.* Your body hears everything your brain says, and it reacts accordingly. And if your brain is full of a lot of stressful and negative beliefs, your body is in a constant state of fight or flight and is merely trying to survive another attack. *Your body, and its trillions of cells, hears everything your brain says.*

This is both concerning and empowering. Science shows us that negative and worrisome beliefs predispose your body to illness; positive and hopeful beliefs are healing and curative. Medical research on beliefs shows us that your beliefs can be self-fulfilling prophecies. One study showed that 79 percent of medical students report developing symptoms suggestive of the illnesses they are studying because of the intense focus upon the illness.[1]

Findings published in the *Indian Journal of Psychiatry* found that our beliefs and our thoughts are neurotransmitters. What this means is that our beliefs create chemical messengers in our brain that communicate information throughout our brain and our body, affecting every aspect of our functioning, including our blood pressure, our immune responses, our sleep, and our digestion. Yes. Take that in. *Your body hears everything your brain says.* In another study, scientists found that "cognitive beliefs could be as potent as pharmacological interventions in terms of modifying biophysical processes in the brain and changing behavior."[2] This last study is proof of what is known as the placebo effect, which is defined as a beneficial effect produced by a placebo drug or treatment that cannot be attributed to the properties of the placebo itself, and must therefore be due to the patient's belief in that treatment.[3] Meaning a doctor can give someone a sugar pill and tell them it's going to heal them, and it does.

Ted Kaptchuk, a professor at Harvard Medical School, practitioner of TOM, and author of *The Web That Has No Weaver*, is a leading researcher on the placebo effect who states that about 60 percent of subjects taking placebos get better, even when they know they're taking a placebo. He concluded that the placebo effect goes well beyond the sugar pill the patient is taking: "Placebo effect is everything that surrounds that pill—the interaction between patient, doctor or nurse. It's the symbols, it's the rituals. These are powerful forces."[4]

In her book, *Everything You Need to Know to Feel Go(o)d,* Dr. Candace Pert describes how emotions and beliefs cause biochemical reactions in both your brain and your entire body. It's as if there is an entire response system in your body that reacts to your everyday beliefs, causing cellular and neurochemical changes. As Dr. Pert says, "You're literally thinking with your body and the words you say . . . which actually affects the neural networks forming in your brain." In other words, your beliefs not only affect your body but also form your body by way of creating and impacting the nerve pathways in your brain.[5]

Penny Sarchet, a researcher who has written about the nocebo effect (which is when a negative expectation of a certain outcome causes a more negative effect than would otherwise occur), explored how a patient's belief in their health and their ability to have hope makes a world of difference to that person's health. Even more, Sarchet stated that what a doctor says and what the patient believes may be more closely tied to the patient's outcome than what the doctor does physically. Studies on the nocebo effect have found that when patients have fears or deep doubts about getting better it has negative health consequences.[6]

When you think a stressful thought or have a belief that makes you feel uneasy or upset, your body reacts at the cellular and neurochemical level. The science shows that such worrisome and illness-focused beliefs actually trigger your brain into its fight-or-flight stress response, dumping cortisol and epinephrine into your bloodstream and causing a cascade of events that render your body more predisposed to illness. This scarily suggests that we can actually think ourselves sick.

On the other hand, thinking positively about your health, believing something out there can help you, having hope, and feeling worthy of optimal health actually has a positive effect on physiology. Laboratory experiments on humans have found that positive moods reduce stress-related hormones, increase immune function, and promote the speedy recovery of the heart after exertion.[7]

A comprehensive review published in the journal *Applied Psychology* found that positive expectations are associated with better health. The review looked at over 160 medical studies and found consistent evidence that a person's positive beliefs are a strong influence for the good on their health.[8] In addition, who you surround yourself with affects your health. Science shows that people who have satisfying relationships with family, friends, and their community are happier, have fewer health problems, and live longer. Conversely, a relative lack of social ties is associated with depression and later-life cognitive decline, as well as with increased mortality.[9]

3) Your Beliefs Are Changeable

Yes! This is the best part about your beliefs! You have the power to change them, and changing your beliefs will change your health. How? Easy. You can change your beliefs by choosing to do so. Really, it can be that simple. What you believe is nothing more than an agreement you have made with yourself about your reality, so to change it all you have to do is change that agreement. To change your beliefs, change the conversation you have been having with yourself and your world. To change your health, it is absolutely vital that you take an honest look at your core beliefs and determine if they truly match your health goals. If you believe you aren't going to be healed, yet you are looking to be healed, you are not in alignment with your health goals, so despite your best efforts healing will likely be difficult. Alternatively, if you are open to the idea that your body can change and heal, then you will allow your brain and your body to transform at the biochemical level.

So, how do we begin shifting your beliefs?
To start, we must first identify what it is you believe.

What Do You Believe About Your Health?

The greatest weapon against stress is our ability to choose one thought over another.

— WILLIAM JAMES, HARVARD M.D. AND FAMED 19TH-CENTURY PHILOSOPHER AND PSYCHOLOGIST

Now that you are ready for healing, you need to assess what your beliefs are, based on how you feel on a daily basis. Before we begin to unpack your health beliefs, I want to remind you that I am not here to tell you how or what you feel is wrong. Rather, I am here to teach you how to reconnect to the innate wellness that is within you, so you can change your beliefs, shift your behaviors, and start feeling better. I know you are ready for a transformation. So let's be real and honest and dig deep into the thoughts you are thinking that are holding you back from feeling better.

I am going to help you identify your beliefs because until we shift your beliefs about your health and your potential to thrive, nothing I recommend will make any difference in your life. You could skip ahead in this book and read about the diet or what supplements to take or how and when to meditate, but *only* when you believe that you can heal and feel better will you begin to see the radical shift in your body's health.

OK. Let's do this. Let's look at your belief systems as revealed by the behavior choices you make about your health every day. Over my 13 years of clinical experience in working with patients, I have zeroed in on four basic limiting beliefs that many of my patients express:

1. "I am my illness." What I mean is that people who define themselves by their illness have handed over their power to their sickness, and wellness will not be available to them until they re-identify themselves. You compromise your health the moment you decide to disconnect from the innate wellbeing that exists within you, and to allow your illness to define you. When you are identified by your illness, it will shape your life. Remember: your body hears everything your brain says. How often do you tell people "I have _____" or "I am suffering with _____ [fill in the blank with your illness or ailment]." If this resonates with you, I want you from this moment on to begin telling your story differently. We are going to get into this more in Chapter 5, but for now you can change your statement to, "I am working on my health. I am starting to feel better." Or, "I may have been told I have _____ but I am no longer letting that define me. I am committed to feeling better."

2. "Nobody feels *that* good." This is another extremely common core belief. Many of you go through life believing things like *This is as good as it gets*, or *No one really feels good* or *Everyone suffers*. While it has some truth—not everyone feels their best all the time—some of you may not even know that feeling better is an option. It is! Wellness is your innate right; feeling well is what your body's default position is. Yet, for some reason you are not there right now. Is it because you don't believe in your body's innate state of health that is your natural born right? If this resonates with you, know that I will help you believe again. For now, start to recognize all the really good, solid health that is around you. Take time to reflect on how your body supported you in the past. Recall a time when you were feeling better, tune into the emotions you felt then, and try to bring them up again. Remind yourself that you did feel well before and you can feel well again. If you can't remember a time when you felt well in the past, think about a time in the near future when you will be feeling better—how you will look, what you will experience differently, how life will be then. We will work on this more, in Chapters 4 and 5 and throughout this book, but for now just start seeing the wellness in your body—past, present, and future.

3. "It's my genetics." Another belief that almost everyone has is that they are destined to get sick because it's hereditary. Does the following statement resonate with you? "My mom/dad/grandmother/ grandfather had _____ [fill in the blank], so I will get it." This is old-fashioned thinking. As we discussed, recent studies show that disease is much less about your genetics than about your epigenetics. The science of epigenetics completely disproves this type of default "It's my genetics" thinking. Less

than 5 percent of diseases are actually inheritable, meaning that only 5 people out of 100 will ever get a particular disease that has genetic links. Instead, your beliefs and how you live your life determine whether the genes for the disease or ailment get triggered or turned on. Believing it's all in your genes has no business being a part of you. You are *not* your genetics. If you think this belief is one you hold, I want you to start noticing all the diseases that people *don't* get that run in their family. I want you to read up on epigenetics. And I want you to know your genes are not set in stone.

4. "I feel bad feeling good." Which can also sound like, "I don't deserve anything better" or "I'm not worth it." Oh, my self-sabotaging sweeties! This belief means that you feel unworthy of feeling better, so you hold yourself back by making lifestyle choices that don't support your health. This type of thinking will absolutely keep you from allowing wellness to fully be yours. For most, worthiness issues are a part of the story, whether it's health or career or relationships. If you see yourself in this statement, know that you are not alone. We will fully address this belief and how to rework it, but if this is you right now, I want you to begin saying to yourself, "I am allowed to feel better" or "I am worthy of feeling good."

The one thing *all* of these core beliefs have in common is what I call *body-disconnect*. Body-disconnect is a loss of connection to the physical, emotional, and spiritual aspects of self, resulting in systemic body chaos. My eczema flare-up on my breast is the perfect example: I was disconnected from myself emotionally, which caused me extreme stress and manifested itself in a physical symptom. It wasn't until I reconnected to myself, and worked through the emotional stress I was putting myself in *because of the belief I had about not being good enough if I stopped breastfeeding,* that my physical symptom was resolved. It's the same with all autoimmune conditions. At the very root of autoimmunity is a cellular misidentification that is based on being disconnected from yourself. Being disconnected from yourself is that feeling that you're keeping a secret and choosing to do something you know you shouldn't. The only person this really hurts is *you*. You are only separating from your self, your wholeness, and your wellness; worst of all, you are standing in your own way. I am not saying you're to blame for your current state of health, but I am urging you to reconnect to yourself so you can heal yourself. I *know* that, if given the choice, you wouldn't choose to be in the state of health you are in right now. I want *you* to befriend *you*.

In order to truly heal and thrive and know what your body needs, you must begin to reconnect with yourself. The pathway back to thriving health lies in tuning in to that internal dialogue going on in the privacy of your mind. It's about hearing and taking note of what you are thinking and believing. You can do it!

Chapter Three

○

The *Body Belief* Pillars

Now that you have a clear idea of what autoimmunity is from both a Western and Eastern perspective, *and* you are grasping the concept that your beliefs play a huge role in your health, it's time to begin your transformation by exploring the three pillars of the *Body Belief* plan. Together, these three pillars have the ability to reshape and resurrect your health:

1. RECONNECT

2. RENEW

3. REAWAKEN

I've been in the business of health and wellness for 13 years, and what I have learned is that the indispensable key to getting someone to take back the power over their health is getting them to realize they actually do have the power to do it. Most people don't realize their power. Most people don't even exercise a fraction of their power. Instead, most people hand over their power to ingrained beliefs that may or may not be serving them anymore. The *Body Belief* plan challenges those old limiting beliefs, and shows you a pathway back to your power. Its guiding principles will teach you how to reconnect to yourself on every level, so that you can renew the beliefs that you have about your body, and from that place begin shifting your behaviors to best support and reawaken your health.

The most necessary pillar of the *Body Belief* plan is to reconnect to yourself. Reconnecting means listening to your body, hearing the conversations you have in your own mind, critically (and lovingly) questioning your beliefs, and getting back to knowing you as you are right now—inside and out. When you reconnect to you, to your body, to your thoughts, to the beliefs that shape your perception of the world, and to your everyday choices, that's when radical healing happens.

When you reconnect to you, you can hear yourself and how you talk to you; you can now understand why you treat you the way you do, and why you choose to do one thing instead of another. When you reconnect to you, you begin to know you better than anyone else, and to understand that you have the power to shift your beliefs and your behaviors. Through reconnecting to yourself, you begin to own the fact that you have the ability to see in a different way the world and how you move about in it.

Now, don't fret, this knowing of yourself is not an overnight thing or a snap-your-fingers-and-it's-done process; it will take time. Be patient and kind with yourself. Start now by saying to yourself, "I know that my body is hearing everything my brain says and I am going to start saying kinder things to myself. I deserve that, my body deserves that." Even if you don't fully believe that statement, say it to yourself three times, right now.

Many people walk around in a state of complete disconnect from themselves. And then they further disconnect by means of vices, like losing themselves in hours of television, social media, a couple of cocktails daily, or codependent relationships. Pick your vice; they all do the same thing—disconnect you from yourself, your situation, your feelings, your pain, and your joy. Listen, we all have our indulgences, and it's not bad to have them. It becomes a vice, a problem, only when you are using them solely to disconnect all or most of the time. Hear me: be easy on yourself. It's OK if you're disconnected right now, because I know you can get reconnected. If I can get you to shift from being disconnected most of the time to being disconnected only some of the time, you will surely see major changes in your health and your life. That one step will bring major changes!

At the very root of autoimmunity is the body not recognizing itself and therefore mistakenly attacking itself. Said another way, your autoimmunity—your body's misidentification of self—can begin to be healed only when you rekindle the relationship you have with yourself. As that reconnection grows stronger, you will honor yourself, you will hear yourself, and you will start the process of renewing your beliefs. Once your beliefs shift, your biochemistry will shift, and from that place the body will stop attacking itself—cellularly and emotionally. This first pillar of the *Body Belief* plan—reconnect—leads right into the second pillar: renew.

Renew means to start the process of shifting your beliefs about your body, your health, and how you function in the world from where you are now to a refreshed version of you. Renewed beliefs are not necessarily different from the beliefs you currently have; they may simply be a more positive variation of them. An example of a renewed belief is transitioning from "I don't think I'll ever feel good again" to "I believe there's a possibility that I could heal." You now know that beliefs and thoughts create chemical messengers in your brain, and when these thoughts and beliefs are activated over and over again, they actually form chemical pathways in your brain. That's why you often hear something like "it takes three weeks to change a habit." Your brain needs to get rewired. So this renewal will be a gradual one, because your brain needs time to adapt to the new belief. You need time to become more comfortable with the new belief.

Your believing the new belief is very important to your transformation. I see it as soothing yourself from a less-good-feeling belief into a better-feeling belief. Slow and steady works better and lasts longer than cold turkey. The ultimate goal is to feel better than you do right now. There will be many more opportunities in this book to renew your beliefs, particularly in Chapter 5. For right now, the renewed belief I want you to start thinking is: *I believe have the power to change my beliefs and radically shift my health.* Which leads us to the third pillar: reawaken.

Reawakening is when you come back to life, where your healing process takes root and the transformation begins. It's where your new tools become habits and your new *Body Belief* lifestyle becomes you. In this book, the reawaken phase is all about what you are going to shift in your diet and your personal care routine to truly amplify your health and wellness. But it's not until you reconnect to you and renew your beliefs that you can really allow for your reawakening. Your reawakening is where the rubber meets the road. To put it all together: *when you reconnect to yourself and your beliefs become renewed you will reawaken your health.*

Each pillar can be achieved only if the one before it has been completed. When you reconnect to your body, you will be able to renew your life by making lifestyle choices that feel good, and your health will reawaken.

Let's look at this process in action. Lisa was a 46-year-old married mother of three children when she came to my clinic for the first time, complaining of pain. She had been a stay-at-home mom for the last 22 years, and as her last child was leaving for college she began to realize that raising three children while her husband worked a stressful, 80-hour-a-week job had taken its toll on her body. As she described it, "The pain is everywhere. Everything just hurts, all the time. I'm on like ten different medications and nothing is helping."

Like many of my patients, Lisa had been to numerous Western medical doctors for her symptoms, and they each offered her a different reason for her pain along with a different medication. Based on reports from these various doctors, Lisa was told she had everything from irritable bowel syndrome to fibromyalgia to endometriosis to chronic fatigue syndrome. She was taking a medication for each of these conditions, plus sleeping pills, daily antacids, and an antidepressant. As I did my intake on her, her symptoms lined up with a typical autoimmune condition: chronic fatigue, whole-body pain, constipation, diarrhea, acid reflux, swollen joints, brain fog, depression, itchy and red skin, insomnia, and extremely painful periods with heavy bleeding and a lot of clots.

I asked her, "How long have you had these symptoms?"

"It's embarrassing to say, but I don't really know. I just know I have felt like crap for at least ten years. I'm just so miserable—can you help me?"

As I asked more questions about the frequency and duration of her symptoms, she couldn't answer me. She had no idea what foods upset her stomach, when her last period was, what made her pain better or worse, what inflamed her skin, what helped her sleep, or even how many hours a night she slept. She was completely disconnected from her body. Moreover, when we started discussing her emotional state, she told me, "I can tell you how my kids feel each day, but I don't know how I feel anymore. I don't know the last time I felt good in my body, but I'm ready for that to change. I'm sick of taking all these pills."

Lisa was completely disconnected from herself. As I do with many of my clients, I took her recovery step by step, with baby steps. First Lisa needed to reconnect and start listening to her body again, so she could know what she felt and believed about her health and her body. Meditation, journaling, and our weekly acupuncture sessions helped her with that. She began to realize that her belief system dictated that once you become a mom, your life was no longer about you; it was only about the health of your family. I worked with her to renew her belief from "It's only about them. I don't matter anymore" to "If I don't take care of myself, I am no good to my family. I am very important." As she began to believe that renewed belief, she started saying "no" more often, rediscovered some hobbies she once loved, rekindled her romantic connection with her husband, and wholeheartedly followed my diet and lifestyle recommendations. And with that, she reawakened her health. Lisa followed the same path you are going to follow: RECONNECT → RENEW → REAWAKEN.

Lisa and I still work together. She has been a client of mine for six years, and over that time she has completely transformed her health and her life. What I helped her realize was that for 25 years she put everyone else's needs before her own. She ignored her own feelings and her physical body for a very long time, and instead of taking care of her body she just took medications. Now she meditates daily, is connected to her emotions and expresses them, and eats the *Body Belief* way. As a result, she rarely ever has stomach issues, and her pain is 85 percent better. She sleeps through the night, has enough energy to do 30 minutes of exercise each day, is happy, has gone through menopause, has lost over 40 pounds, and only takes the medication of an occasional sleeping pill when she's stressing over one of her kids. She told me recently, "Before I met you I thought this is what aging feels like, you're supposed to just feel like crap. You're supposed to take all this medication. I was resigned to the thought that being a mom meant you take care of your kids and no one else. Now I know I am worthy of taking care of me and that I have so much power over my health and my well-being."

When Lisa first started seeing me, she wasn't connected to her body. She had no idea why she was feeling so unwell. As we worked together, she began to listen to her body, to the conversation she was having with her body; and she slowly began her health transformation.

You too can transform your health. You can reconnect to you and your body, you can renew your beliefs about your health and your body, and you can reawaken your health by making choices from a place of *knowing* your body. You can step back into your power and take care of the most important person in your life, YOU. That is the *Body Belief* way.

It all begins with you forming a kinder, more loving, more compassionate, and more supportive relationship with yourself. Reconnecting to yourself allows you to see the beliefs you have and how they are affecting your life. Once you can see those beliefs you can decide to change them. And in that moment, you are taking back the power over your health.

RECONNECT → RENEW → REAWAKEN

It's really that simple.

Now, take a deep breath, let this new way of seeing your health and your life sink in, and let's get into how you are going to start your reconnecting process.

Chapter Four

○

Reconnect to You

Reconnecting to yourself is the most important pillar of the *Body Belief* plan, because what I have found is that most people who walk through my clinic doors are like Lisa: They are disconnected from themselves. They are not in touch with their current state of health—mentally, emotionally, physically, and nutritionally. They don't even have language for their emotional space beyond "I'm doing OK." And they can't quite convey their physical symptoms. It's like they're in a fog.

They may have a medical diagnosis they received from a Western doctor before coming into my office, such as Hashimoto's thyroiditis, rheumatoid arthritis, eczema, or endometriosis, but beyond that they don't really know how they feel or how to listen to their bodies. For instance, about 80 percent of the new clients I meet don't know whether or not they had a bowel movement that day, or what it looked like, or how it felt coming out. Most of them are not sure if they feel rested in the morning, or how they feel after a big meal, or if they have more or less mental clarity as the day progresses. And if I were to ask them about their emotional space, most of them would not connect to that either. In fact, when we start discussing what it is they feel, they can't really figure it out. They can identify what they are feeling only superficially, but not why or how long they've been feeling it, or from where it really stems.

In order to transform your health and heal you must be able to connect and communicate with your body, and it must be able to connect and communicate with you.

Do you ever connect the dots between your actions and how you're feeling? For instance: "I skipped breakfast and had only a large cup of coffee; maybe that's why I feel so lightheaded and my heart is racing." Or, "I have such a headache in the morning; maybe I was clenching my jaw all night in my sleep because I'm so worried about _____ (fill in the blank)." Or, "I feel so short-tempered and frustrated all day; maybe it's because all I do all day is take care of everyone else and I have no time to take care of myself."

What I would love for you is something like this: "I slept eight solid hours last night, and I feel so clear-headed today." Or, "I ate a healthy breakfast this morning and my energy levels are better than I can remember." Or, "I meditated for five minutes today and I feel so grounded and present."

Many people lack effective communication with their body and mind. They have very little body awareness, and their emotional clarity is less than ideal too. What I am going to teach you is how to listen to your emotional and physical body cues so you can go from wondering "Why do I feel this way?" to "I know how I am feeling and why." You are going to learn how to reconnect to you so you can heal.

The word *reconnect* means to connect back together, to reestablish a bond. I am going to help you reestablish kind and compassionate communication with your body—from your cells on up. Your healing depends on it. Remember, autoimmune disease is a result of confusion and miscommunication in the body; something that was once identified as being part of you is now being perceived as something that is foreign and that needs to be rejected. It's as if your body's GPS can't find a cell signal to get directions back home. There's a loss of communication, a dropped signal, a cellular amnesia. Even more, it's not just cellular miscommunication that causes your immune system to attack cells that are healthy and normal—it's your emotional disconnect too.

Take Jennifer, a 38-year-old stay-at-home mom. She came to my clinic two years after the birth of her second child. I asked her how she felt and why she was coming to see me, and she said, "I feel like I've been hit by a truck." When I asked her to describe her symptoms to me in more detail, she couldn't. All she could tell me was how tired she was. Only when I began asking specific questions like, "What are your bowel movements like?" or "Do you have any skin rashes or dryness in any area of your body?" could she give me more information. As I completed my intake, I discovered that she experienced diarrhea, constipation, extreme fatigue, headaches, skin rashes, cold hands and feet, hair loss, terrible brain fog, depression, and joint pain. When I asked her about recent blood tests that her doctor took, she told me, "My thyroid is normal."

"No. Something is definitely up with your thyroid," I said.

I have been practicing long enough to know exactly what a thyroid condition looks like. When I looked at Jennifer's lab results, her thyroid numbers were within the normal range for the lab tests but they were not in the functional range. There's a big difference: normal on a lab test can be a lot higher or lower than what a healthy functional range should be. (We will cover what the ranges should be in Chapter 9.) So I suggested that she get a few additional tests. Sure enough, the new blood work showed what I suspected: Hashimoto's thyroiditis, an autoimmune condition of the thyroid where the immune system begins attacking the thyroid gland. Her doctor told her that medication wouldn't help her at this point and perhaps she should talk to an endocrinologist. Frustrated and confused, she came back to me for a plan to get her health back. She wanted to feel better immediately.

What happened with Jennifer is a very common scenario: she sought help from her doctor, but unfortunately didn't know what questions to ask. The doctor only did cursory blood work that didn't give a full enough picture for a proper diagnosis. When I work with my patients, I always attempt to work in tandem with Western medical doctors to get my clients back on track. Very often, I have to urge my patients to go back to their doctors and ask for more tests that will be more thorough and give a fuller picture of what is going on.

Western medicine is very unclear about the treatment and diagnosis of autoimmunity, and therefore these conditions are often misdiagnosed or, even worse, the patient is told it's all in her head! Studies show that most autoimmune patients see a handful of doctors before they get the correct tests done. I try to help streamline that process as much as I can by informing you on all the lab tests (and their functional ranges) that you need to have your doctors do, plus many tools so that you know the right questions to ask your doctors.

Your health is in your hands, and it's your right to advocate for yourself as part of that!

"Tell me what to eat. Tell me what vitamins to take. I'll do it all—just help me feel better," Jennifer said.

"I will do all that," I said. "But there's still so much more for us to talk about. . . . Tell me about your emotional state. Are you happy?"

She started to cry. "Of course I'm not happy. I feel like crap every day."

"When was the last time you were happy?"

She paused. "I don't know."

"So, were you happy before you started feeling unwell?"

"I guess not. Life's just been so hectic with the kids, and my husband hates his job, and we're so stressed about money, and I miss working. I'm so exhausted all the time and impatient. I really don't like myself or who I have become. It's all too much. Is there a vitamin for that?" she joked through her tears. "Really, it's that I don't even know who I am anymore."

I handed her a tissue. "I hear you."

The truth is, I hear this all the time. Especially from women who are suffering with autoimmune conditions. What I have concluded is that not only is there a loss of connection on the cellular level, but there is one on the emotional level too.

Take Jennifer, for instance: Yes, she has an autoimmune thyroid condition that is causing her physical ailments, but what about her emotional mind-set? She confided in me her complete state of unhappiness, how disconnected she feels from herself, how she doesn't even know who she is anymore. Her feeling unwell physically is just one piece of what is going on with her, and it's completely tied to how she is feeling emotionally. What I discovered with Jennifer, as I have discovered with hundreds of other clients, is that the emotional piece preceded the physical symptoms.

Why?

Because her body heard everything her brain had been saying.

Jennifer's brain was saying, "I don't like myself or who I have become; I don't know who I am anymore."

And then her cells started saying the same thing: "Even though you were once a part of me, I no longer recognize you, so I am going to attack you." That's what autoimmunity is—a state of being disconnected from yourself so much that you can no longer differentiate self from the non-self, cellularly or emotionally.

What I saw in Jennifer is something I see often, even in myself—an inability to connect the dots as to why they feel the way they do. Take the example about myself that I shared with you earlier about the eczema I had from the emotional turmoil I was putting myself through over stopping breastfeeding. So many of you are doing the same thing I did—you are not living in your body enough of the time to understand the *why* behind how you are feeling. Maybe you have constipation but don't understand why—is it from what you're eating, your stress levels, dehydration, or all of the above? Or are you short-tempered and have fits of rage but aren't clued into what sets you off or who or when the next attack of rage is coming? Or do you have incredibly restless sleep because you go to bed with so much on your mind that you spend the whole night processing instead of resting? This disconnection comes from moving through life too fast to notice the reason things are happening, and usually people move so fast precisely because they are avoiding their connection to their hearts and minds and bodies. They have numbed themselves to all feeling, and that cannot go on too long without ill effects.

So, are you disconnected from you?

Do you feel like you don't even know who you are anymore? Are you constantly judging yourself, blaming yourself, angry at yourself in your mind? Are you still lamenting a decision that you made days, months, or even years ago? Are you not pleased with yourself for the current state of your life? Do you no longer like who you see in the mirror? Do you feel like you are an outdated version of someone you once knew?

If so, you could be doing more harm than good to your body.

There are two ways to disconnect or separate from unwanted parts of yourself: you can disconnect either with love or with hate. When you separate from unwanted parts of yourself with hate, that's what I call *hostile disconnect*. Hostile disconnect is a state of angry self-rejection where you tend to be very unkind to yourself and your body—for example, by abusing your body with alcohol, overeating sugar, not exercising, or ignoring unpleasant feelings like rage, unhappiness, sadness, or grief. Hostile disconnect creates the breeding ground for autoimmunity. On the contrary, when you disconnect from unwanted parts of yourself with love, I call it *kind disconnect*. And it's just that: kindly deciding to let go of parts of you that no longer serve you. When you disconnect with kindness you are choosing to nourish your body, mind, and soul by listening to its cues; you are changing course for the next phase of your life. You might be ending a relationship because it gives you more pain than joy, leaving a job where the environment is toxic, or giving away the skinny jeans from college that haven't fit you in 15 years.

How do you know if you have a hostile or kind disconnect? The best way to tell is to look at how you view others, how you interact with your environment, and how you treat your body. The actions you take regarding these three categories are a reflection of how you feel about yourself.

If you don't think your anxiety, depression, sadness, and stress impact your physical health, think again. All of these emotions trigger chemical reactions in your body, which can lead to inflammation and a weakened immune system. Learn how to cope, sweet friend. There will always be dark days.

— KRIS CARR, WELLNESS ACTIVIST AND *NEW YORK TIMES* BEST-SELLING AUTHOR OF *CRAZY SEXY DIET*

Think about it: when it comes to other people in your life, are you judging them harshly? Do you feel they are always doing it wrong? What about your environment? Do you honor your home environment and its contents? Do you treat your property and your belongings with respect? Do you dress with a sense of pride? And when it comes to your body, do you respect how much it does for you on a daily basis? Do you choose to give it the nutrition, rest, and fuel it needs to thrive? Do you live in it enough to be aware of how you feel after each meal or upon waking? Take a moment to reflect on this and be very honest with yourself. Do you look out into the world and see compassion and kindness and love and hope and potential? If so, then that's what you see in yourself. But if you look out into the world and see doom, danger, and malicious intentions, then that's a reflection of what you see in yourself, which sets the stage for self-rejection and disconnect on every level—mentally, emotionally, and cellularly.

I am not here to judge you or to have you bring judgment upon yourself. Rather, I am here to bring awareness to how you are being kind or hostile to yourself, your environment, and your body. It is in this awareness that you can transform. When you reconnect to the truth that lives within you, you can begin to live from a place of self-love, compassion, and kindness.

If you're feeling defensive right now, or concerned about your connection with yourself, that's totally normal. Many of us are disconnected from the core of who we are and how we really feel. In today's world it's fairly easy to disconnect. The media, your mobile phone, your vices, your relationships, your to-do lists—they can all distract you and disconnect you, severing ties with who you really are and how you really feel. In order to get through the day emotionally intact, you may have learned to live more in your head and less in your body. Maybe your job has hardened you some, or the noise of the city you live in has detached you from being present, or the home you were raised in wasn't a very connected one so you weren't ever shown how to connect to your body.

Body Belief Exercise: Instant Reconnect

Here is a quick and easy reconnection tool you can start using *now*. Take in a long, deep breath right now and ask yourself, "_____ (fill in the blank with your name), where are you?" This is something I do in my life *all the time*. Especially on my busy work days when I'm seeing clients back-to-back and feel like I'm moving so fast I'm leaving my body. I stop (usually at the sink when I'm washing my hands), take a deep breath, and ask myself, "Aimee, where are you?"—only to realize I am paying more attention to whether I am running on schedule than to my patients' needs. Or maybe I'm thinking about how I have to pee but I don't have the time for it right now. Or I'm already thinking about heading home for the day. Asking myself this one question brings me right back to the present moment and to my body. Just the act of asking yourself this question helps you reconnect, because it brings you from wherever you are mentally to being back in your body.

For instance, right now you are reading this material and taking it all in, but chances are you are also going over all the things you may be doing in your life that disconnect you. You may be thinking about the past or future, clenching your jaw or tensing your shoulders, or beating yourself up in your head. Whatever it is, taking a moment to tune in to yourself and get back in touch with where you are will help you begin the reconnection process. Use this tool whenever, wherever, and as often as possible.

Reconnecting to your body, forgiving it, and showering more kindness and love upon it will help you rekindle your relationship and reestablish open lines of communication with it, so that you can heal. As one of my most trusted spiritual teachers, guru and *New York Times* best-selling author of *Return to Love* Marianne Williamson, has said, "Enlightenment is a shift in perception from body identification to spirit identification. You become unstuck because it becomes less about you." My interpretation of this is that you are living too much in your head and not enough in your heart. In TOM, we say the heart is where your spirit resides. When you are living in a state of disconnect and self-rejection, your spirit shuts down. You become spiritless, lacking excitement or drive or ambition. You are just going through the motions rather than living with zest and liveliness. This is the misidentification of self. This is where you lose you. You want to be happy, you want to feel alive, you want to be giddy about life. And you deserve to be.

You may be wondering, "What does any of this have to do with my Hashimoto's diagnosis or my rheumatoid arthritis or my celiac sprue or my psoriasis?" It has everything to do with it, since it is not until you are connected back to the core of you, open to your spirit being enlivened, feeling worthy of thriving health, that you can truly receive it.

It all starts with you living in your body again; with you shifting from a place of hostility to one of compassion. Your body— and all the cells in it—hears everything your brain is saying. What you say to yourself, you say to your cells, and to your body as a whole. Your physiology shifts in response to what you say. If you are still mad at yourself for something, or blaming a situation for how you feel, you are not allowing in forgiveness and compassion. You are in hostile disconnect. That conversation in your mind needs to shift from one of hostility to one of compassion, because your body hears everything your brain says. This isn't about suddenly being happy and optimistic 100 percent of the time—that's unrealistic. But this is about being kind and compassionate and gentle with yourself, more than you're not. It's about reconnecting more than you're disconnecting.

What does being reconnected look like?

I see reconnecting as this idea of getting back in touch with who we are. Being reconnected means living in your body, not just your head. It means feeling what's going on, tuning into how your body reacts to the foods you eat, the situations you're in, the emotions you feel, the things you are saying to your body consciously and unconsciously. This involves experiencing pain but also joy. You cannot have one without the other, and in order to reconnect to you, you will feel it all. And that is a good thing! Disconnection usually happens because of pain—something in your life caused you pain, and instead of dealing with it, you shut it out. The reconnection lies in going through the pain and healing from what hurt you. When you allow yourself to move through the pain and the discomfort, you begin the reconnecting process, and you open up to allowing joy to fill the space of the pain. When you reconnect, you slow down, you begin to hear yourself, you begin to talk back to that inner voice with compassion and forgiveness. Eventually, when you're more reconnected than not, you have a presence of mind to easily and confidently state your feelings and your needs. You react less and listen more. You feel aligned with life, like things are working out for you the way they should. You trust the process and how things are unfolding. And most importantly, you take full responsibility for how you feel, for where you are, and for how your life is, because you know from your place of reconnection that you have the power to positively influence and shift your life and your health. Doesn't that sound nice?

Autoimmunity is a cellular attack against the self. It's the body's attempt to destroy and eradicate other parts of your body. It's hostile and angry. Love and kindness is the antidote. Belief in your body is key. Cheering yourself and your cells on is imperative. Finding peace with where you are and feeling worthy of all you desire is where transformation can take place. This isn't about perfection; this is about being easy on yourself a little more than being hard on yourself. If you got to a point where you were kind to yourself more than you're not, you will see some major transformations in your life. You're going to get there because you are worthy of feeling better.

Get Mindful

There's all this talk about being mindful, but what does being mindful even look like? Let's define that through showing you what's *not* mindful. You're not mindful when you skip breakfast and don't understand why you have zero energy to get through the day, or when you are dealing with a bad breakup and your back goes out and you don't see the connection, or when you want to speak up at work over a miscommunication but instead you stifle your feelings and get a major stomachache. You are mindful when you listen to the cues your body and your mind are giving you. Being mindful is realizing things like, "I have a headache because I am so stressed about _____ (fill in the blank)." Or, "My stomach is aching because I don't want to fight with _____ (fill in the blank)." Or, "I am ignoring my grumbling stomach. I know I'm hungry, but it can wait." Or, "I am still so pissed at my ex for leaving me that I'm only going to date people who can't really ever commit to me."

Yes, being mindful allows you to get deep with yourself. It allows you to reconnect with you, to begin to understand the *why* behind your actions and where you are in your life. The best way to get more mindful is to slow down enough to hear what your mind and your body are saying. Your body hears everything your brain says.

Here are some of my favorite tools for becoming more mindful.

Tool #1: Sit and Breathe

Your new priority and your first tool is to start hearing what it is your brain is saying.

You're going to do this by adopting a daily meditation practice. I know meditation can be scary, but it doesn't have to be. Starting to meditate doesn't mean you have to completely upend your life or move to a monastery in Tibet; it just means taking time to slow down, feeling your lungs fill with air, and being a part of each inhalation and exhalation. It's about reconnecting to you. One simple way to do that is a quick meditation:

1. Set a timer for three minutes. You can use a smartphone, a meditation app, or an egg timer; they all work.

2. Find a comfortable and quiet place to sit or lie down. Don't stress about how you're sitting or lying down; there is no right or wrong here. You don't need a special mat or socks. Really, you just need to be comfortable.

3. Close your eyes.

4. Breathe. Yes, really! Just breathe.

5. Take in a nice comfortable three- to four-second inhalation and a nice comfortable three- to four-second exhalation. To keep your mind off of racing thoughts, count during your inhalation and exhalation. It goes like this: Inhale, one, two, three, four, exhale, one, two, three, four. Continue this cycle until your timer goes off. And if a thought comes up, that's OK. It's not about being without thoughts while you're meditating; it's more about letting them pass by without attachment.

That's all there is to it. Sure, meditation can get more intense, or you could choose to use a mantra or buy a special candle or a special outfit. And if you want to do all that, go for it. But you don't need anything special to quiet your mind and just breathe. Make it your goal to get mindful every day for a few minutes (if you skip a day, that's OK; just make sure to get back to trying it out).

Sukha Purvaka Pranayama (a.k.a. easy yogic breathing)

If you want to try something even more therapeutic with your mindfulness practice, try pranayama breathing. *Pranayama* is an ancient yogic practice that controls the breath to enhance vitality and life force.

Here is a basic pranayama breathing exercise for inflammation and relaxation:

Instructions: Sit comfortably on the floor or a firm chair with your eyes closed and spine straight. After several natural breaths, inhale slowly and deeply for six counts into the belly, ribs, and upper chest. Exhale slowly for six counts from the upper chest, ribs and belly. Do this simple breath for four to eight rounds. If you feel uncomfortable, you can reduce the count to four. This should be easy and relaxing. Rest after your practice of one to two minutes.

Physical benefits: opens up the lungs, keeps the mind calm, improves digestion, and relieves fatigue

Why meditate? Over the last 10 years, hundreds of scientific studies have been released on the benefits of meditation. Here are some of the noted effects of a regular meditation practice:

- Increases immune function
- Decreases pain
- Decreases inflammation at the cellular level
- Increases positive emotions
- Decreases depression, anxiety, and stress levels
- Increases social connection and emotional intelligence (meaning it helps you reconnect to your emotions)
- Improves the ability to be compassionate
- Changes your brain for the better
- Improves your memory
- Increases focus and attention
- Increases productivity[1] (yes, by sitting still and breathing you will become more productive!)

You see, meditation helps on so many levels. Most importantly, what a regular practice offers you is the ability to reconnect with you, so you recognize your thoughts and observe them rather than react to them. Think of meditation as flossing—you don't always want to do it, but you know you should. If you don't floss, your teeth, gums, and oral hygiene will suffer and cause you pain. If after seeing all the ways meditation can transform your life, the idea of sitting still and breathing still feels challenging, try this: take a little extra time in your daily bath or shower to get in 5 or 10 long deep breaths. Start there, and as you get more comfortable with that habit, try the meditation practice I discussed above.

A few common beliefs that stop people from meditating are:
I don't have enough time
It feels selfish
I'm too anxious to sit still
It doesn't work for me

To all of those excuses, I say: If you want your health to thrive, be open to the possibility of change and the benefits you can receive from taking time each and every day to breathe and slow down. Meditation isn't about perfection. It's about you prioritizing you because you know you deserve it.

No excuses, just breathe!

Tool #2: Listen and Take Notes

As you begin to slow down on a daily basis and get more mindful, you will inevitably begin to hear more clearly the conversation you are having with yourself in your mind. Whether it's in a journal or a text message or an e-mail to yourself, I want you to begin to tune in to the following and write it out:

1. ABOUT ME: What are the regular things you worry or stress about? What makes you feel frustrated or angry on a regular basis? Write out as many things as come up.

2. ABOUT OTHERS: How are you judging others in your head? What do you say to yourself about others when you see them on the street or in the office? Are you saying kind things or not-so-kind things? Write out as many things as come up.

3. ABOUT MY SPACE/MY ENVIRONMENT: How are you treating your environment? How do you leave your home when you head out for the day? Do you make your bed or straighten up the kitchen? Do you leave trash on the sidewalk or in your car? Do you fold your clothes and put them away or just throw them on the ground?

4. ABOUT MY BODY: How do you treat your body? What do you say about your body when you look in the mirror? Do you dress yourself with a sense of pride? Do you even look at yourself in the mirror?

5. ABOUT MY FEELINGS: How do you feel during your day? Take at least three check-ins each day and write down the emotions you are feeling in those moments. Write down the first emotion that comes to mind.

Stuck? Here are some common emotions that you can use to describe how you are feeling:

Happy	Irritated	Enraged
Sad	Open	Confident
Alive	Annoyed	Good
Bitter	Calm	Resentful
Excited	Lousy	Peaceful
Ashamed	At ease	Powerless
Fortunate	Guilty	Thankful
Tense	Grateful	Upset
Free	Embarrassed	Spirited
Skeptical	Loving	Alone
Anxious	Hopeless	

This is another exercise in mindfulness. There is no right or wrong here. All I want you to do is begin to see yourself and take note of it. No judgment here, just honest reflection. Doing this exercise on a regular basis will help you begin the reconnection process, and it will help you a lot when we get to work on renewing your beliefs. So get yourself in the habit of practicing your meditation for several minutes and then afterward spending a few more minutes taking notes on where you stand in relation to yourself, your judgment of others, your space, your body, and your feelings. As always, there is no right or wrong here—all I want is for you to begin to understand how you work, think, feel, and believe.

Tool #3: Say Something Kind

Did you know that 70 percent of everyone's subconscious thoughts are negative? I bet you are regularly say things to yourself like, "You can't do that," "That will never happen," or "I'm not that lucky." Now that you are becoming more mindful, and taking note of the things you are saying to yourself and how you are interacting within your world, I want you to begin the process of responding to your inner dialogue with kind words. For example, whenever I am rushing around because I am running late for something (which, for a very long time, was very common for me), I say to myself, "You always do this to yourself, Aimee. When are you going to learn? Why do you always wait until the last minute? Haste makes waste, and this is why you're always screwing things up." In my more mindful days, when that conversation happens, I now retort with something like, "It's OK, Aimee. You are constantly learning more about yourself and you are better at this than you once were. It's OK, Aimee. I love you just the way you are."

Here are some examples of kinder things you can begin saying to yourself when you catch yourself in that not-so-nice internal dialogue:

I am in the process of learning more about myself, and I am getting better at it all the time.

I am doing the best I can from where I am right now.

I love you. It's OK.

Be easy on yourself, _____ (fill in the blank with your name).

I am reconnecting to my body and finding more ways to be kind to myself, and that feels good.

Pick one or more of the above statements that feel good to you and start using them. Your body hears what your brain says, and using some of these kinder statements will help remind your body that you support it and love it. I know that if you have stayed with me this far, you are serious about reconnecting to yourself, so give yourself a pat on the back for all that you are doing for *you*.

This process should be a slow and steady one; it's not a switch you can flip from off to on. Be kind to yourself in the unfolding of your reconnection. All I ask of you is to take time to breathe more, listen to that conversation in your head, take a few moments each day to use the Instant Reconnect tool (p. 40), and be patient with yourself. Chances are, you are not going to like all the things you hear in the privacy of your own mind, and you might not see the connection between your thoughts and your physical symptoms, but I know you will begin to. So hang tight and be more of a cheerleader for yourself than not. If you succeed at that, even just 70 to 80 percent of the time, you are making some amazing progress.

OK, take a deep breath, send some love to the trillions of cells in your body (I'll do the same because our cells deserve it!) and turn the page so we can dig even more deeply into what you believe about your body and how it affects your health.

Chapter Five

Renew Your
Body Beliefs

I began working with Melissa when she was 33 years old. She was engaged to be married to a man she loved, but she was also working 80 hours a week in a dead-end job, sleeping only 4 hours per night, living on a diet of Diet Coke, fat-free cookies, egg-white omelets, and the occasional vitaminwater. She was a super anxious and overwhelmed person who spoke so fast I could barely keep up during our first meeting in my clinic. She came to me after being diagnosed by her urologist with interstitial cystitis, a common autoimmune condition, with symptoms of urgent, uncontrollable urination. She was following a course of treatment recommended by her Western medical doctors, but it wasn't helping. She was desperate for something that could help her feel better. A friend of hers urged her to see me.

Melissa didn't know anything at all about Traditional Oriental Medicine, but was at the point where she would try anything to feel better. As I did my intake with her, asking her questions about her lifestyle, her emotions, and her physical symptoms, I realized there was a lot more going on than just her urinary issues. She was an insomniac, sleeping way less than four hours a night, had terrible digestion—she was gassy, bloated, and constipated most of the time—and had frequent skin rashes, daily headaches, nearly constant heart palpitations, heavy and painful periods, and pain with sex, which left her with no sex drive. And on top of everything else, she wholeheartedly believed that her condition was the result of a past sexual relationship.

A few years back, she was in a relationship with a man she loved, but she discovered he had been cheating on her with a lot of different women. She broke it off with him, but ever since then she was convinced she caught an STD from him, and truly believed that he and his cheating were the cause of her current symptoms. Even though all of her STD tests were negative and the doctors had diagnosed her as having an autoimmune condition, not a bacterial or viral illness, she couldn't shake the feeling that he had caused her current vaginal and urinary medical troubles; and worse yet, that she had given her illness to herself by being with him.

Melissa told me she had recently started seeing a psychotherapist, because she was obsessively thinking about the actions of her cheating ex and she feared her emotional state was going to impact her current relationship. Over the course of several treatments, Melissa shared a lot with me, revealing a deep resentment toward the cheating ex-boyfriend, anger at herself for ignoring the signs that he was cheating, overwhelming shame over what had happened, a distrust of men, and a nagging fear that her current fiancé would also cheat on her. She admitted she hated her body. She was disgusted by it, and felt she had betrayed it by sleeping with a cheating, dirty ex-boyfriend, and that she deserved to be suffering from her symptoms.

Melissa clearly had a lot of negative beliefs about her body stirring around in her head. The treatment plan I devised for her was as much about lifestyle changes as it was about emotional introspection, self-forgiveness, and shifting her beliefs about her body and what it deserved. As she began to reconnect to her body (using the "Listen and Take Notes" tool on p. 47), renew her beliefs about her body, and forgive herself for the past, not only did she start to feel good about her new diet and supplement routine, but she started sleeping better, her anxiety quieted, and her urinary and vaginal symptoms dramatically improved.

She has since gotten married, regulated her periods, birthed two children, and remained off all her Western medical treatments for her condition, since it resolved without the need for further medication. Through my guidance and tools, the work we did together, and the help of her psychotherapist, she has become aware of her body, her emotional state, and the interconnection between her emotions, her beliefs, and her health.

Melissa now understands that her belief that she should have some sort of physical discomfort or repercussion for having been with someone who cheated on her was exacerbating, if not creating, her symptoms. The only time she gets a flare-up of her urinary symptoms is when she's under moments of extreme stress, during which she is being really hard on herself about not being good enough, or feeling shame about something she did or didn't do. Thankfully those times are rare, and when she does go there, meditation, journaling, psychotherapy, and creating a kinder dialogue with herself alleviates her symptoms.

Does any of Melissa's story resonate with you? Do you see a correlation between a traumatic event you experienced—like the death of a loved one, a bad breakup, the loss of a job—and when your physical symptoms began to appear? Do you see a flare-up in your red-flag symptoms (the ones we discussed on p. 10) under times of stress? Do you find yourself saying things like, "With the way I have treated my body, it's no wonder I feel this way." Or, "With what I have been through, my body could never bounce back." Or, "I deserve this because of _____ (fill in the blank; typically the first thing that pops in your head is the thing)." If you felt even a slight pang of a "Yes" answer to any of the above questions, know that with the help of this chapter (and this entire book) you will be able to shift and renew your beliefs so you can get beyond what is standing in the way of your wellness.

A word on psychotherapy...

Before we move any further, I want to tell you that digging deeply into our beliefs and our emotional lives isn't always easy, but it's always worth it. Even though it can be difficult and challenging, I believe in you. I know you can do this, and I know you are willing to. Now is the time to begin healing ourselves, to forgive ourselves, and to see that there is another way. If you feel you need more emotional support and guidance beyond this book, or you want to really get to the bottom of any traumatic experiences in your life, seek professional help from a psychotherapist. Therapy is a very good thing, and can really be the help you need to make the changes you want in your life. It can help you make the connection between thoughts and behaviors, come to terms with past traumas, or simply get unstuck.

What you believe about your body and its health is at the root of how you talk to it, how you interact in your world, and ultimately how you feel; and all of these factors create chemical messengers in your brain and influence how your body works on the cellular level. *Your body hears everything your brain says.* All of the fifty thousand thoughts you have each day influence how your body functions. Don't fret too much, since one of the best things about your beliefs is that *you* can change them. How to change and RENEW your health beliefs is what we are going to focus on in this chapter.

Let's use the thought that was at the root of Melissa's physical condition as an example: "I deserve to be suffering because I'm not good enough." Somewhere in the aftermath of Melissa's finding out what her cheating ex did, she began to blame herself for his actions. Chances are this belief of hers was longstanding, and the incident with her ex triggered it. Whatever the case, Melissa's thought process went something like this: my ex cheated on me because I wasn't enough for him; my body wasn't good enough for him; I must be unlovable; I deserve to suffer; my female parts deserve to suffer. She blamed herself so deeply for her ex-boyfriend's failings that she punished herself and her vagina for his misdeeds.

Her behaviors and life choices shifted to support and perpetuate that repetitive, wholehearted belief. She worked 80 hours per week, barely slept, ate poorly, and hated her body. And her whole vaginal area became inflamed! From her chronic belief that she deserved to suffer, Melissa's behaviors supported that belief *and* her brain responded to that stressful belief in a stressful way—by creating inflammatory chemical messengers in her body, rendering her body in an autoimmune deficient state. The good news: Melissa changed her beliefs, optimized her health, and created a new positive relationship with every part of her body—and *you* can too.

If you're thinking, "There's just no way my thoughts and my beliefs can have an impact like that on the cells in my body," think again. Scientific research clearly shows that trauma and/or consistent stress has the "capacity to underlie the later development of physical disease by chronically stimulating stress neurocircuitry, neurohormones and proinflammatory cytokines. The intensity of the stress response is more important to an individual's neurobiological response than its nature."[1] Did you catch that last part? *The intensity of the stress response is more important to an individual's neurobiological response than its nature.* What that means is that stress and negative thoughts have a greater influence over your health than your genes. It's more about epigenetics—how you nurture your body, or don't—that influences whether those genes are turned on or off.

In Melissa's case, her beliefs were causing or exacerbating her urinary symptoms. In my case, the belief that others would consider me a bad mom if I stopped breastfeeding at nine months caused my eczema to flare up on the body part I needed to use for breastfeeding. The manifestations of both Melissa's and my symptoms—in her vaginal area and on my breast—are not coincidental; in fact, in TOM they're diagnostic.

In TOM, we are trained to examine where on the body an illness manifests, and then look deeply into the emotional aspects of that body part, area, or organ. The energy pathways that run through the body correlate with different organs, and each organ has a physical *and* an emotional component. For example, when someone complains of lower-back pain, I am trained to look at what could be going on physically in the region of the lower back; but I also look into the emotion associated with that area. TOM associates the lower back with the kidney organ, and the kidney is linked with the emotion of fear. So I'll always talk to patients about any possible fears that they are experiencing in their life. What I see with back pain or a back going out is that it often comes up during a time in their life when they have a fear of a big decision in their life. It's as if they are believing the thought, "I am afraid to move forward on _____ (fill in the blank with any decision)," and their body hears it and says, "OK. I will make you immobile so you have some more time to think about this," or "I'll lay you up so you don't have to make the decision you're afraid to make."

If we look at Melissa's case, the area where she was experiencing her symptoms was the female reproductive system. There are a few different energy pathways that run through that area, but in combination with our intake and her history it became clear that she was hating her female parts, particularly her vaginal area, because they were causing her not only physical, but also emotional, pain.

Something similar happened to me once: I had an emotional pain connected to a physical symptom in a very telling place on my body. When I was 27 years old, I was engaged to a man I loved, but some part of me also knew he wasn't right for me. Still, I said yes when he proposed, and I wore my engagement ring with pride as I began planning our wedding. As the months went on, I began to develop one of the worst cases I have ever had of eczema *on my left hand* (the same hand I wore my engagement ring on). I tried everything to make it go away. I talked to every kind of health practitioner, and uprooted my diet and changed all of my supplements. But the eczema wouldn't budge. One day I was talking to my acupuncturist, who knew my body and my emotional state extremely well, and she said, "Do you think that maybe you have an aversion to being engaged? And your body is responding with this screaming, red, itchy, painful skin condition?" She was absolutely right. When I broke the engagement, the eczema went away, never to return on that hand again (though it did return to my breast; clearly, eczema is one of my red flags that pops up when I'm not being true to myself).

In TOM, we don't see the mind and the body as being separate. They are connected; they are one. In order for whole-body healing to take place, the mind and the body must be taken into account. And that is why right here, right now, we are going to start working on *you* renewing your body beliefs!

Renewing Your Beliefs

Renew means to start the process of shifting your beliefs about your body, your health, and how you function in the world from where you are now to a refreshed version of you. But let me ease you some—I am talking about taking current beliefs and shifting to a more positive variation of them. There's no way anyone could go from a place of feeling "I feel like crap every day" to "Everything is sunshine and rainbows and chocolate." That's not real life. I am talking about small, consistent, real-world shifts, like going from "I feel really unwell most days" to "There's a chance I could feel better." Or from "There's no hope for me" to "I felt a little better today for an hour, so maybe there is a light at the end of the tunnel." Or from "It's my genetics, I'm just built this way" to "This epigenetic stuff is really interesting; I wonder what I might be able to do to turn things around in my body." The renewal I want you to experience is a *gradual* one, because your brain needs time to adapt to the new belief, and you need time to get comfortable with your new way of thinking.

Tell me: Do you think your stress levels, or your chronic negative thoughts, or the thoughts you have about your body might be having an impact on your health? Back in Chapter 2, I brought up the four most common beliefs I see in the clinic that deter thriving health:

1. I am my illness
2. Nobody feels *that* good
3. It's my genetics
4. I feel bad feeling good

Do you identify with any of those statements? Are you cheering yourself on, or verbally abusing yourself? Do you believe that you are worthy of thriving health, or that you deserve to suffer? Do you think optimal health is attainable, or something that few have? If autoimmunity is the self attacking the self, are you attacking yourself? This is a big question, I know. But you've come this far, so I know you are ready to hear me; I know you are ready to shift from where you are to a better-feeling place, and changing your core beliefs is what is going to get you there. Listen, this isn't a simple process, and it can take months, sometimes years. But if you want to achieve lasting change in your life and in your health, identifying and renewing your beliefs are going to get you there. And even if at this moment you don't fully believe in your ability to make these changes, I believe in you. I know you can renew your beliefs. I have seen hundreds of people do it, and you can too.

We are not seeking perfection here. We are seeking ease. We are trying to find better-feeling beliefs than the ones you currently have. If you can start thinking better-feeling beliefs a little more often than not, change will happen.

Tool: The A.R.T. of Shifting Your Beliefs

Now that you have reconnected with yourself, and hear what you are subconsciously saying to yourself, I am going to show you how to retrain your brain to renew and shift your body beliefs. Your perception of your health can transform your health, in either positive or negative ways. It is time to Acknowledge, Renew, and Transform (A.R.T.). With this tool, I am going to give you back the power over your beliefs and how they are influencing your health.

You will use this tool to acknowledge your fear-based, health-hindering thoughts, so that you can then renew them into kinder, more compassionate, and more loving thoughts, which will then truly allow you to transform your health and your life. The *key* to getting the most out of this tool is honestly witnessing the thoughts (your beliefs) that are limiting you. The transformation lies in your ability to be open to the idea that shifting your beliefs can make a difference in transforming your health and your life.

Your thoughts dictate your behavior, and your behaviors dictate your health (and your life!).

ACKNOWLEDGE: The absolute best way to begin to *acknowledge* your thoughts is to tune in and reconnect to you. By this I mean to really *listen* to that internal dialogue, what you are saying to yourself in the privacy of your own mind. And then when you hear those sneaky thoughts (and you will!), write them down here so we can begin to work them out. Go back to the tools I gave you in the last chapter and use them to help you acknowledge what it is you currently believe about your body.

To get you started, I am going to list some common health-thwarting beliefs. These all stem from the four that I discussed on p. 58. Put a check next to any one of them that resonates with you:

I've tried everything to feel better, but nothing works.

☐ I always knew I would get sick.

☐ I'm too old to change.

☐ I'm set in my ways.

☐ There's no hope, so why bother?

☐ I have bad genes; it's in my blood.

☐ I'm afraid to feel better.

☐ I don't know who I am without my illness.

☐ I'm afraid to do this alone.

☐ I'm not sure I believe that my body can heal itself.

☐ I'm reading this book because someone told me I should, but it won't work for me.

☐ My doctors said there's nothing they can do to help.

☐ My doctors said I will never be healed.

If you identified some of your own fear-based, power-sucking thoughts that I didn't touch upon, fill them in here:

_____

_____

_____

_____

_____

RENEW: OK, now that we have acknowledged some of your limiting thoughts that don't serve you (or your health), let's begin the work of renewing those thoughts. Renewing your thoughts is not about going to the complete opposite thought. For example, going from "I feel like crap every day" to "I am the healthiest I have ever been and I'm walking on sunshine" would be a big, unrealistic stretch. Rather, renewing a thought is just finding a better-feeling thought. It's like going from the thought of "There's no hope" to "I suppose something could work for me." All I want you to begin to do is soothe yourself with a better-feeling thought. If you need more help than this exercise, bring your questions to our *Body Belief* Facebook group and I will help you reform your thoughts. For now, try some of these renewed thoughts and see if they resonate with you. The way you'll know if the thought works for you is you will feel a sense of relief or ease. Put a check next to the ones that give you that sense of, "Yeah, it does feel better to say it that way":

- [ ] I do feel better when I take better care of myself.

- [ ] I want to believe that I can be healed.

- [ ] I am ready to feel better.

- [ ] I know stress affects my sleep, so I guess it could be affecting my overall health.

- [ ] There are a lot of people going through health challenges like mine.

- [ ] If I really think about it, I am not alone in this process.

- [ ] I have read about how other people radically changed their health.

- [ ] There does seem to be a lot of science supporting the epigenetics theory.

- [ ] I suppose there's no harm in making the dietary changes Aimee recommends.

☐ I have never fully committed to all the recommendations Aimee makes; I could try them and see.

☐ Aimee has helped thousands of women optimize their health; I could be one of them.

☐ Doing the emotional work Aimee suggests can't hurt.

☐ I know in my heart I am meant to feel better than I do now.

☐ My body is programmed to thrive, I just need to properly support it.

If you identified some of your own better-feeling reforming thoughts that I didn't touch on, fill them in here:

_____

_____

_____

_____

_____

_____

TRANSFORM: Good for you for making it this far, and really digging into and breaking down those limiting thoughts. Now, the key to transforming your health (and your life) is saying to yourself the renewed thoughts when the fear-based, power-sucking thoughts come up. You can do this in the privacy of your own mind, out loud, or in a journal—whatever works. Get into the habit of talking lovingly to yourself. For instance, if you're having a bad day, you might say to yourself, "What's the point of all this? I am still not feeling good!" If that happens, it's OK. The true transformation lies in what you say back to yourself: "AHA! But, I do feel better than I did last month!" You are still going to have moments when you say not-so-nice things to yourself. All I am asking you to do is respond to yourself with a renewed and better-feeling thought, such as "I am doing the best I can do. I have incorporated a lot of changes and I do feel better. Patience isn't easy, especially with this whole process, but I am getting better."

Use the space below to write out some kind, loving thoughts to yourself and then take them to our *Body Belief* Facebook page and share. Your words may help someone else on their path to healing.

_____

_____

_____

_____

_____

_____

_____

By getting to the core of what you believe about your health, and what you say in the privacy of your own mind, this A.R.T. tool is the foundation of thriving health.

I know we just went deep on the emotional front, and I'm sure you're still processing it all. You may even be wondering if this is right for you. The A.R.T. tool may take some time to digest and get used to. In the meantime, I have a few more exercises that I think can really jumpstart a renewal of your beliefs.

Tool: The Feeling Tracker

I want you to go back to p. 10, where I had you check off which red-flag symptoms you were experiencing. Now I want you to pick the *top* three to five symptoms from that red-flag list that affect your life the most. In a notebook or a journal, write down these top symptoms, so that we can rate them in a few different ways. At the top of the page, write down the first symptom and then create four columns beneath the symptom, labeling the columns as follows: How I feel, How I want to feel, Why, and What's holding me back. It'll look something like this:

ECZEMA

How I feel	How I want to feel	Why?	What's in my way?

For the first column, using a scale of 1 to 10, rate the symptom (1 is no symptoms and a quiet body, heart, and mind; 10 is every symptom fully raging, yelling, and screaming). In the next column, use the same scale and write down how you want to feel.

I want you to take a moment and imagine what it would feel like to experience the number in the second column. What would it feel like to be at a one or a two . . . or a zero? Would your body feel less tense, would you feel more free—or would you feel more rested, more social, and less depressed? From this imagination exercise, gather your thoughts and write out in the "Why?" column why it is you want to feel better than you do. Next, take a moment and reconnect to yourself and see if you can tune in to what is in your way of getting to that better-feeling place. Identify the belief that is preventing you from getting there. Often I find that patients are held back by the first belief that pops into their mind after writing down the "Why?" The mental conversation often goes like this:

"I want to feel like a two."

"Why?"

"Because I will have more energy to do what I want to do; I will feel more clear-minded."

And then the bully inside their head steps in with the negative body belief, and says something like, "I've tried everything to feel better, but nothing works." Or, "There's no hope, why bother?" Or, "I'm too old, this is what happens with aging." This exercise is super powerful because you are now getting in touch with *why* you want to feel better, as well as recognizing the belief that needs some renewing. Eventually you will get to a point where, when you hear the negative belief, you won't believe it anymore. In fact, you will be able to talk back to that bully inside your head with a renewed belief. And that is when your transformation really begins!

I recommend doing this practice daily, or even several times each day. It will get to the point where you don't need to write it out; but I still think you should at least write out your "Why," so you will see it change on a regular basis. Taking the time to really visualize and feel the "Why?" behind why you want to feel better will help you get there.

Tool: I Am . . .

One of my favorite tools for renewing beliefs is sort of a fake-it-till-you-make-it kind of thing. I want you to take one or more of the below statements, and in your journal or notebook, write it out 10 times (or even better, 100 times!).

I am strong

I am healthy

I am healing

I am kind to myself

I love who I am

I forgive myself

I can hear my body and what it's telling me

I appreciate my body

I honor my body

I have hope

After you have written down each statement, I want you to get in front of a mirror, look into your own eyes, and say the statement out loud. Say it at least 10 times. Be warned: this exercise may make you cry or feel tense, or it may bring up unexpected emotions. Let them come up. Be kind to yourself. This is a wonderful tool to open yourself up to the belief that things can get better. Practice this as much as you can and come up with some of your own statements that make you feel good when you write them or say them out loud. I want you to eventually find ways to weave these "I Am" statements into your everyday conversations and interactions. For example, when someone asks you, "How are you today?" you respond, "I am hopeful." Or, "I am feeling healthy."

Tool: The Good Journal

We're adding a lot of things to this journal of yours! This exercise doesn't actually have to be done in a journal; you can do it via e-mail (to yourself) or on your smartphone (in a notes app). What I want you to do is notice what is good in your life; notice what is working. We go through our day thinking subconscious thoughts that are mostly negative, so let's respond to them with some positivity. Each day, or several times per day, take some time and write out what feels good for you—even if it's something as simple as, "This chair I am sitting in feels good." Or, "Taking the time to write out what feels good, feels really good." Or, "The sun is out today and that feels good." Keep it simple: don't overthink this. Just write out at least five things each day that feel good to you.

The act of doing this will allow for more kindness and love in your body; it will outweigh the hostility and allow your cells to heal. Training yourself to notice good things, no matter how small, is an easy way to begin renewing your beliefs from a place of hopelessness to a place of hope.

OK, I have given you a lot of tools to work with, so you can renew your beliefs and take charge of your health transformation. Since your body hears everything your brain says, be kind, compassionate, and easy on yourself. You are an awesome human being, and the world is lucky to have you. Own that truth. Even if you own it only 70 to 80 percent of the time, you are headed in the right direction. Even if you are being kind to yourself only 70 to 80 percent of the time, you are shifting your physiology and the cells in your body are healing. Even if you are reconnecting to yourself and working on renewing your beliefs only 70 to 80 percent of the time, you are on the path to radical healing.

I do not want you to aim at getting perfect at this, because there is no such thing as perfection, and seeking perfection will make it easy for you to find ways to be hard on yourself. Rather, be flexible, be open to change, be willing to see things differently, be willing to believe in hope again. This process is about retraining your brain, not about achieving some state of everyday euphoria. Life is going to happen, you are going to have slip-ups, and you are going to have days when you will be hard on yourself.

That's OK. Just use the tools I have given you, and tune in to your-self so you can hear when you are being hard on yourself and respond with some kindness and love. You deserve that much.

Take a deep breath and give yourself a big hug, because we just laid the groundwork for you and your renewed beliefs—*and that's a big deal.* When you're ready, head into the next chapter, where we are going to get into all the nutritional and lifestyle changes you can make for thriving health.

Chapter Six

Ｏ

Reawaken Your Health

Here you are, armed with amazing information on how to reconnect to yourself, so you can hear the conversation you are having with your body and its cells in the privacy of your own mind. Couple that with all the tools you now have to help yourself renew some old and stubborn beliefs that are limiting your ability to heal and thrive, and you are so ready for your reawakening! When I talk about reawakening your health, I am talking about bringing your health back to a state of optimal functioning. At its core, your body has an innate knowledge of wellness and vitality; wellness is its default position. We are going to reawaken that wellness and reboot your system back to a state of feeling good more than not.

In this chapter, we are going to cover a lot: from why food is the best medicine that exists, to what to eat, to what not to eat, to the only cleanse and purify your healing body will ever need, to what supplements to take, to how to rid your home from toxic chemicals, to how you should prepare your food, to mindful mealtime practices. There is a ton of information in this chapter that you are now ready to take in, because you are reconnected and renewed, and your body is now open to receive its reawakening. I am excited with how far you have come, and I can't wait for you to have the health you long for. You so deserve it!

To help you understand why the dietary changes laid out herein are imperative to your healing your autoimmunity, I want to revisit two things we have previously discussed:

1. The three vital substances in TOM: qi, blood, and essence

2. Leaky gut syndrome

As I mentioned in Chapter 1, according to Traditional Oriental Medicine theory, when it comes to resurrecting your health, qi, blood, and essence are supremely important. Qi is the building block of life and the core of health and vitality; it is life force. The number-one place we get our qi from is the foods we eat, and the number-two place is the air we breathe. When it comes to food, we have a saying in TOM: "If it sits on your counter and it doesn't go bad, don't eat it because it has no qi."

Qi is found in foods that are as close to their natural state as possible, such as lush, organic green spinach, or bright orange organic sweet potatoes, or farm-fresh pastured eggs with the most golden yolks you have ever seen. In contrast, food that comes in a package with food colorings, pesticides, high-fructose corn syrup, and synthetic vitamins has no qi. Examples include processed spinach pies, microwavable sweet-potato fries, and egg-replacer that comes in a box. Make sense?

There's a lot of food available to us, and an enormous variation in the quality of that food. For five thousand years, Traditional Oriental Medicine has preached the necessity of eating a diet full of life-giving, nutrient-dense, and qi-rich foods that maximize overall health and vitality, and improve the quality of each and every of the 37 trillion cells in your body. That's what we are after here—reawakening all the cells in your body so you can radically heal. Eating qi-rich foods will fill your body with an abundance of qi, which lends itself to vibrant and reawakened health. Alternatively, a shortage of qi will leave you feeling exhausted, achy, foggy headed, cranky, constipated, and unwell.

Now that you are reconnected to you and are working on your renewed beliefs, the you that you know and love again deserves food that is packed with qi. When you regularly eat qi-rich foods, your body can take the nutrition from those foods, creating healthy blood and essence. And when it comes to dealing with autoimmunity, all three of these substances (qi, blood, and essence) are vitally important to your healing.

When the body is full of qi, blood, and essence, the organs will work properly and the person will be healthy or, at the worst, might suffer only minor and short-term diseases. Alternatively a deficiency of qi, blood, and essence allows environmental factors to affect the body, such that the autoimmune disease will progress and become a serious illness.

Bottom line: the food you eat and the amount of qi it has impacts every single cell in your body. I am going to teach you what to eat so you can best support your health, nourish your vitality, and maintain an abundance of qi, enabling you to heal.

Now let's discuss leaky gut and how it's involved in autoimmunity. About 80 percent of your immune system is in your gut, and that's why healing your gut is imperative to healing your autoimmunity. Think of the lining of your digestive tract as a fishnet stocking with extremely tiny holes that allow only very tiny and specific substances to pass through, keeping out bigger particles. A healthy digestive tract doesn't let any unwanted particles into it. Even though there are holes in it, they are tiny and extremely particular as to what they let in. But when a person has a poor diet (filled with foods that have no qi, or life force), is under a lot of stress, or is exposed to environmental toxins (emotional and physical), the holes in these fishnet stockings become bigger and less particular about what substances pass through them. This is when the gut becomes leaky and allows proteins, bad bacteria, undigested food particles, or toxic waste to enter into the digestive tract, where they don't belong. When leaky gut, or increased intestinal permeability happens, it sets off an immune reaction in your system.

Even though these food particles, waste, and protein are in your body, they are not supposed to be on the other side of that highly particular fishnet stocking. Once they are, the immune system attacks, because they are foreign substances for that part of the body. When the immune system engages and attacks these foreign invaders, it sets off systemic inflammation, aggravating your entire body and leaving you with symptoms like bloating, fatigue, joint pain, headaches, skin rashes, acid reflux, diarrhea, constipation, gas, depression, anxiety, and muscle pain. Basically all those red-flag symptoms we went over back in Chapter 1 can happen when the gut becomes leaky.

The Western medical-research consensus is that leaky gut must be present for autoimmune diseases to occur.[1] What that means is that if you are regularly experiencing a handful of the red-flag symptoms we went over, or have been diagnosed with an autoimmune condition, it is highly likely that you have a leaky gut. But just as your beliefs can change, your leaky gut can be repaired, and I am going to show you how.

Just as foods with no qi leave your body deficient in blood and essence, and render you unwell and prone to chronic disease, so does leaky gut. The good news: you can change both of these by upgrading your diet to nutrient-dense, wholesome organic foods that are as close to their natural state as possible. Food is the best medicine that exists, and I am going to walk you through everything you need to know about it, show you how to implement a healthy diet, and cheer you on as you allow the foods you eat to help you heal.

To Diet or to Detox

I want to talk to you about something very important: diets and detoxes. Those two words make me cringe because they are fads; they are not sustainable. Every day of your life should be a detox—meaning, it's imperative that we all eat a nourishing diet that is free of toxins most of the time. The *Body Belief* plan is not a 30-day diet or a 7-day detox (there is a PURIFY phase in the *Body Belief* plan, but rest assured you can eat real food during this phase!). The *Body Belief* plan is about shifting your entire lifestyle—mentally, emotionally, physically, and nutritionally—so you can reawaken your health and maintain that state of health. Doing a 4-day juice detox or a starve-yourself crash diet isn't going to bring lasting changes to your health. **Making a commitment to changing your lifestyle—on every level—is the only thing that is going to give you the thriving health you deserve.** Yes, really! Commit to yourself. You are the detox, you are the diet, it's in you!

The *Body Belief* Eating Plan

Now that you have a better understanding of how the food you eat impacts your health and your autoimmunity from both a TOM and a Western perspective, I am going to walk you through the *Body Belief* eating plan. But before we get into all the details, I want to remind you of something that is very important: be easy on yourself. The recommendations that follow may at first be overwhelming to you. Don't let that deter you. Take baby steps if you need to. Spend more time in the PREP phase (you'll see what I mean in just a moment) or circle back to the PURIFY phase when you feel more mentally prepared for it.

Even if you begin just with cutting back on the foods I say not to eat, that's a great start. Of course, if you want to see radical changes in your health and autoimmunity, committing to the entire plan, written out as is, will get you there the fastest. But you can ease yourself into it. For some of you, these changes have already begun. For others, all of this information is brand new.

Wherever you are, know that it's exactly where you're supposed to be. So, be easy on yourself, start making changes that feel comfortable to you, and use your red-flag symptom tracker to guide you.

As you begin seeing your symptoms improve, you will feel more and more encouraged to continue on this path and incorporate all of the plan recommendations. I promise you that by committing to the entire plan, you will be cultivating healthy and abundant qi, healing your leaky gut, and supporting your immune system so that your autoimmunity can heal. Plus, you'll find that you will sleep better, move better, have glowing skin, have shiny hair, have strong nails, and feel vibrant and alive in a way that you haven't in quite some time. This is *your* body and *your* healing process; there is no right or wrong as long as you are being kind to yourself while making lasting changes to your lifestyle. Use the shopping lists and menu plans I have for you on my website, and engage with others in the Facebook group, as there are thousands of women in that group going through exactly what you're going through. So share your journey, listen to others, and get the support you need on your path to optimal health. If it feels right, enlist friends and family members to make these changes with you. Most importantly, *believe* that you can do this and *know* that you deserve the thriving health you desire.

OK, let's get into the *Body Belief* eating plan.

Chapter Seven

○

The *Body Belief* Eating Plan: Framework

The most important tenet of the *Body Belief* eating plan is that all the food you are eating must be high-quality food. By that I mean it's qi-rich, vitality-cultivating, nutrient-dense food that is organic (except for where I have noted otherwise) and non-genetically modified (non-GM), and comes from a humanely raised, free-roaming, pasture-raised, grass-fed, hormone- and antibiotic-free, grazing-animal source. Add to that fresh and local, and you are on your way to truly reawakened health.

Doing the *Body Belief* plan on a budget

I know that this lifestyle overhaul may be a strain on your budget, so I've created this budget cheat sheet so you can make this plan work for you financially.

- **Use coupons:** Local health food stores and even large chain stores like Whole Foods have a weekly coupon guide (Whole Foods even has an app where you can download coupons). Many companies give away coupons on their social-media pages, so follow them on Facebook and Instagram and snag their special deals. You can even go to websites like OrganicDeals.com and AllNaturalSavings.com to find coupons from different companies and retailers.

- **Prioritize:** Animal products are the most important foods to get organic (and grass-fed/pastured) because the commercial versions of these products are the most toxic to you. Next, coffee (if you drink it) is really important to get organic. For all your fruits and vegetables, use the Dirty Dozen guide from EWG.org to prioritize which of your foods *must* be organic.

- **DIY:** Make as much of your own food as possible. From your bone broth to your snacks and meals, DIY and save. This book is loaded with amazing recipes; use them.

- **Buy in bulk:** Buy your favorite products in bulk and save. Many online retailers and large chain stores sell foods and products in bulk at a discount.

- **Skip Starbucks:** Allow more money for your health transformation by skipping your daily Starbucks habit (make your own coffee or tea at home) or any other habit you have that you can replace with something homemade.

My easy-to-follow plan is designed to smoothly transition you into your new way of nourishing your body and its cells. Here's how it is broken down: The *Body Belief* eating plan starts out with a PREP phase, which will ideally last a week (that may be too short for some of you and too long for others, so go at the pace that feels the best to you). In the PREP phase, you are going to start cutting back on certain foods, getting into the mode of cooking most all of the food you eat, beginning to shop for high-quality foods, and mentally preparing yourself for this new way of eating. I want you to take as long as you need in this phase. Knowing how long you need will require you to use your reconnecting skills from Chapter 4 so you can tune in to what your body needs.

The second phase of the plan is the PURIFY phase, where I am going to jump-start your body and its cells with 11 days of eating very simply and very clean—mainly nourishing and satisfying bone broths, soups, and tasty side dishes that are going to boost your qi and begin your healing process. It is not a juice cleanser or starvation diet that will leave you famished and irritable. Rather, it is meant to do two things: to help rid your body of inflammation and any other toxic buildup, and to begin the healing of your leaky gut. Fully healing leaky gut can take months, even years, but you can do it. After you finish up the 11 days of purifying your body, you will move into the REAWAKEN phase, where you will start adding more of the *Body Belief* foods into your diet and evaluate how your body responds. This phase can and should last for the rest of your life.

I have set the *Body Belief* eating plan up this way because it is very important that you eliminate certain foods over a period of time, so that you can determine how your body reacts to such foods. There are many different types of foods that can aggravate autoimmune conditions, but once your immune system begins to regulate itself your body will become less reactive to such foods. Our goal is to find out what your body is most reactive to, so that you can modify this *Body Belief* eating plan to best suit your thriving health. There are some foods that I am going to tell you never to eat again, and there are other foods that I want you to remove from your diet for a few weeks and then slowly and moderately add back in, so you can gauge how your body and your red-flag symptoms react. Since you are now reconnected to you, that will be easy for you to decipher. This new way of eating is going to reset your immune system, slow down or even reverse your aging process, and leave you feeling like a brand-new version of yourself. It is the ultimate topper to your health transformation.

The Food*stuffs* You Should Never Eat Again

I know I just told you that I want you to be easy on yourself and take all this in at your own pace, but I do have to point out some of the extremely toxic and nutrient-depriving food*stuffs* you may be eating that you need to stop eating immediately. Notice, I used the word *foodstuffs*—that was intentional. That's because the following substances I am about to discuss are not actually food.

They offer your body zero nutrition, and they have no business being in your healthy and thriving body, ever.

Gluten

Gluten is the protein found in wheat, barley, and rye—so that means bread, pasta, and beer. Research shows that gluten is the main culprit when it comes to leaky gut and autoimmunity, in particular for those who have a genetic susceptibility to autoimmunity.

When you eat gluten, it triggers the release of a chemical called zonulin, which causes the holes in your intestines—those tiny fishnet-stocking holes—to open up and let in toxic particles, proteins, and other substances that aren't supposed to be on the inside of your intestines.[1] Now, you may want to say to me, "My doctor tested me for celiac disease [CD] and I don't have it." And to that I say, "It doesn't matter." It doesn't matter for a couple of reasons. Although it is estimated that about 1 percent of the population has CD, 1 in 30 people have a gluten sensitivity and about 99 percent of them are undiagnosed.[2] Moreover, eating gluten is linked to malabsorption, which causes a deficiency in your body of many necessary nutrients, such as iron, folate, and vitamins D and K, all of which are essential for optimal health and vitality. Lastly, the gluten protein looks like other tissues in your body, including your thyroid tissue, as a result of which eating gluten will exacerbate your autoimmune condition. (This is known as molecular mimicry, and it happens with dairy proteins as well.)

With all that said, regardless of whether you have celiac disease, you can no longer eat gluten, because it is inflammatory and activates autoimmunity in your body; plus, eating it will compromise your ability to digest and absorb nutrients from *any* foods you eat. Also, all nonorganic wheat products (the most common to contain gluten) are heavily sprayed with toxic pesticides, which have also been linked to autoimmunity. Therefore, in light of the current research, I strongly encourage you to avoid consuming any gluten, organic or not. Even a small amount of gluten here and there will aggravate and inflame your body, and your immune system will attack your precious tissues and organs.

Here is where gluten hides out in the foods you eat:

Barley	Beauty products
Broths (store-bought)	Bulgur
Communion wafers	Couscous
Einkorn	Emmer
Farina	Farro
Graham	Imitation meats
Kamut	Marinades/sauces
Matzo	MSG
Processed meats	Rye
Seitan	Semolina
Soy sauce	Spelt
Stock cubes	Textured vegetable protein (TVP)
Triticale	Wheat
Wheat germ	

As you can see, gluten is pervasive, so when you avoid it you have to avoid all of the above foodstuffs as well.

Can I Ever Eat Gluten Again?

The current science suggests that gluten is most damaging to people who have a genetic predisposition to autoimmune diseases. But with autoimmunity growing to epidemic proportions, we all may soon have a genetic predisposition to autoimmunity. My recommendation is this: Avoid gluten as much as you can, preferably 100 percent of the time. Commit to the *Body Belief* eating plan for at least six months. If you are feeling almost 100 percent better, then, if you must, try some gluten—but be sure it is organic; preferably, it should also be sprouted. If any of your red-flag symptoms recur, consider that gluten might be the culprit, and that leaving it completely out of your diet for good would be best for you. No matter what the science is currently showing, in my clinic I see that most everyone feels a lot better when they avoid eating gluten.

Soy

Soy and its derivatives can be found in virtually every packaged food on the market (soy oil can even be found in many of your vitamin supplements), and you need to stop eating it. Soy products, organic or not, are so overly processed that they are actually indigestible, toxic, and a potent source of xenoestrogens (a.k.a. plant hormones), which have a remarkably strong effect on the hormones within your body. The American Nutrition Association released a thorough review of the currently available scientific literature about soy, which shows it to be a hormonally disruptive antinutrient,[3] meaning that when you eat it, it actually takes nutrients from your body. Although organic, fermented, and non–genetically modified soy *in very moderate amounts* can have some health benefits, I strongly recommend avoiding all processed, nonorganic, and non–genetically modified forms of soy.

Upwards of 70 percent of all packaged foods (even the ones in health food stores) contain soy and soy derivatives, so be sure to read your labels and avoid foods with any of the following ingredients:

Hydrolyzed soy protein
Hydrolyzed vegetable protein
Soy flour
Soy oil
Soy protein isolate
Textured vegetable protein (TVP)
Vegetable oil (this is usually soy oil)

Skip these common soy foods as well:

Soy cheese
Soy milk
Soy yogurt
Tofu

Added Sugars

Basically, when you eat a food with an "added sugar," *even if it's natural and organic*, it causes inflammation throughout your body, exacerbates leaky gut, and causes your blood sugar levels to spike, which in turn causes your body to release insulin to try to regulate and balance your now-high blood sugar level. This puts your body into fight-or-flight mode. And guess what all of that does? It sets the stage for autoimmunity. So read your labels and skip the added sugar!

The common names for added sugar are:

Agave nectar	Brown sugar
Cane crystals	Cane sugar
Corn sweetener	Corn syrup
Crystalline fructose	Dextrose
Evaporated cane juice	Fructose
Fruit juice concentrates	Glucose
High-fructose corn syrup	Invert sugar
Lactose	Malt syrup
Maltose	Raw sugar
Sucrose	Syrup

Artificial Sweeteners and Food Chemicals

Artificial sweeteners and food chemicals are chemically derived and have been shown to have toxic effects on the body,[4] and have been scientifically linked to such diseases as cancer, Alzheimer's disease, multiple sclerosis, and lupus.[5] Since these foodstuffs are chemicals and *not* food, I am advising you to avoid them, forever.

Common names for artificial sweeteners and food chemicals that you need to avoid are:

Acrylamides
AmnioSweet
Artificial and natural flavors
Artificial food coloring
Aspartame
Autolyzed protein
Brominated vegetable oil
Canderel
Carrageenan
Cellulose gum
Cyclamate
Equal
Guar gum
Maltitol
Mannitol
Nitrates and nitrites (unless they are naturally occurring)
NutraSweet
Olestra
Phosphoric acid
Saccharine
Sorbitol
Splenda
Sucralose
Sunett
Trans fats
Xanthan gum
Xylitol
Yeast extract

The goal with the *Body Belief* eating plan is for you to eat foods as close to their natural state as possible, which really limits your consumption of any processed, packaged foodstuff that contains any of these artificial sweeteners and food chemicals.

Exceptions to the Rule: Soy and Added Sugars

As with most things, there are some exceptions to this *never-eat-again* rule I have just given you. When it comes to added sugar, you can have some *in moderation*. That means no more than 10 grams or 1 teaspoon a day. And for soy, if you are a vegetarian or really like soy products, you should be eating only organic, non-GMO and sprouted or fermented soy products (like miso). Still, consume no more than 3 ounces a week. But that said, cut added sugars and all soy out while committing to the *Body Belief* plan herein. Just as with gluten, if after six months following this plan you are feeling almost 100 percent better, play around with adding these foods *in moderation*, and in the allowances I just mentioned.

Processed Vegetable Oils

Once upon a time you were told that vegetable oils and margarine were better for you than things like butter or lard. This stemmed from the theory that vegetable oils, although highly refined and chemically processed, were lower in cholesterol than the fat found in butter or lard and would therefore reduce the risk of heart disease. That cholesterol theory has since been disproven, many times over.[6] Even more, vegetable oils are now known to be proinflammatory—meaning they cause inflammation in your body—because they are high in omega-6 fatty acids.[7] The *Body Belief* eating plan is all about you lowering your omega-6 exposure and increasing your omega-3 intake. Consuming more omega-3 fatty acids in comparison to omega-6 fatty acids significantly increases your risk of developing heart disease, diabetes, cancer, and autoimmune disease.[8] Plus, these vegetable oils are highly processed and refined.

Avoid all of the following, all of the time:

Canola oil	Corn oil
Cottonseed oil	Margarine
Palm kernel oil	Peanut oil
Rapeseed oil	Safflower oil
Shortening	Soybean oil
Sunflower oil	

OK, now that we have gotten those foodstuffs that you are never to eat again out of the way, I want to go over some additional foods that you are likely eating but that have been proven to negatively affect autoimmune conditions.

The Foods That Don't Support Your Autoimmunity

The following foods have all been scientifically proven to exacerbate inflammation and autoimmunity. I want to go over them with you so you can understand why and how they are affecting your body and its cells, and so you can feel good about eliminating them during certain phases of the *Body Belief* eating plan. (Don't fret: later you will get to add these foods back into your diet to see if they feel good with your body).

Dairy

There is a big difference between conventional, grain-fed, pasteurized, hormone- and antibiotic-pumped dairy products and those from grass-fed, hormone- and antibiotic-free cows; but either way, dairy is not super friendly to anybody already dealing with inflammation and autoimmunity. It contributes to leaky gut, is very difficult to digest, increases mucus production, contains lactose (of which almost 25 percent of Caucasians are intolerant), is a cross-reactor with gluten (meaning that people with gluten intolerance will likely become intolerant to dairy), and contains hormones that are linked to an increased risk of cancers.[9] So, with all that said, dairy—especially conventional, factory-farmed, and non-fermented dairy—should be avoided if you have an autoimmune condition. The *Body Belief* eating plan allows you to try adding dairy back into your diet later on. For now, you are to avoid all of the following:

Butter
Butter oil
Buttermilk
Cheese
Cottage cheese
Cream
Curds
Dairy protein isolates
Heavy cream
Ice cream kefir (from dairy; coconut kefir is fine)
Milk
Noncultured ghee
Sour cream
Whey
Whey protein isolate
Whipping cream
Yogurt

Legumes

These foods are members of the pea family, and are commonly known to us as beans. The issue with this class of foods is that the part we eat is actually a seed, and a seed by nature is indigestible, as a plant's means of survival. Let me explain: A plant's mission is to pass on its genes, but because a plant cannot move, it relies on animals and forces of nature, like wind, to spread its seeds. Thus, the seed is highly protected and made to withstand being broken down or digested by any animal that eats it. When you ingest foods that are difficult or *impossible* to digest, inflammation in your body ensues. What makes the legume indigestible is twofold:

1. Toxic lectins: Lectins are found in many foods, but it's the toxic lectins, namely agglutinins and prolamins, that aggravate autoimmunity, increase intestinal permeability, and create systemic inflammation in your body. On top of all that, genetically modified toxic lectins are even more inflammatory than their non-GM counterparts. But here's the catch: these toxic lectins aren't toxic enough to cause you to be severely ill right after eating them. It's more about the chronic exposure to these toxic lectins that can cause or exacerbate inflammation and autoimmune disease in your body.

2. Phytates and phytic acid: These substances are found in all plant-derived foods—seeds, legumes, grains, and nuts—and like toxic lectins they inhibit digestion. In moderation, phytates and phytic acid don't cause major issues, but when you are consuming many foods that contain these substances, your body will become inflamed, your gut will become leaky, and autoimmunity will worsen.

At some point after the inflammation in your body has subsided and you are beginning to feel better, you can try adding soaked and sprouted legumes back into your diet; but for now I want you to avoid legumes in all forms:

Alfalfa	Beans (all varieties)
Carob	Chickpea
Clover	Field pea or garden pea
Lentil	Peanuts
Soybeans	

Grains and pseudograins

We have already talked about the reasons you need to avoid gluten, ideally forever, but for now I want you to also avoid *all* grains and pseudograins, for the same reasons you are to avoid legumes: toxic lectins, phytates, and phytic acid. In addition to all of the gluten-containing grains, here is a list of the nongluten grains and pseudograins that you need to avoid:

Amaranth	Buckwheat
Chia seeds	Corn
Job's tears	Millet
Montina (Indian rice grass)	Oats
Quinoa	Rice (brown, white, and wild)
Sorghum	Teff

OMG! What can I actually eat?

I know I am telling you not to eat *a lot* of foods. But remember, this is for the short term, not forever. So hang in there with me a little longer, and I promise there are plenty of good, yummy, delicious foods you *can* eat!

Nuts and seeds

Nuts and seeds pose the same issues as legumes, grains, and pseudograins, as they, too, are plant-derived and contain toxic lectins, phytates, and phytic acid. As with the other foods on this list, you will most likely be able to enjoy them again (soaked), but for the initial phases of the *Body Belief* eating plan, I want you to avoid all nuts and seeds, including:

Almonds
Cashews
Flax seeds
Hemp seeds
Pecans
Pistachios
Pumpkin seeds
Sunflower seeds

Brazil nuts
Chestnuts
Hazelnuts
Macadamia nuts
Pine nuts
Poppy seeds
Sesame seeds
Walnuts

You also need to avoid any flours, butters, oils, or other products derived from nuts and seeds.

Nightshades

This type of vegetable is the least well tolerated by autoimmune patients and anyone with inflammation in their body. Like grains, pseudograins, seeds, nuts, and legumes, nightshade vegetables contain toxic lectins. They also contain two other substances—saponin and capsaicin—that make them aggravating to the immune system. Saponins have been shown to lead to leaky gut[10] and they contain a substance that both stimulates and aggravates an immune response.

Basically, when you eat nightshade vegetables, your immune system gets more agitated and is more likely to host an autoimmune reaction. Capsaicin acts like a steroidal stimulant when ingested, and although there can be some benefit from such side effects, capsaicin could also further contribute to leaky gut and intestinal permeability.[11] These foods seem to be highly aggravating to anyone with inflammation and autoimmunity, so this is the last food group you can reintroduce on the *Body Belief* eating plan. For now, and maybe forever, you need to avoid the following nightshade vegetables:

Ashwagandha
Bell peppers (sweet peppers)
Cayenne peppers
Curry mixes (the ones that contain any of these nightshade
   vegetables or seasonings)
Eggplant
Goji berries
Hot peppers
Naranjillas
Paprika
Pepinos
Pimentos
Tamarillos
Tomatillos
Tomatoes
White potatoes (sweet potatoes are OK to eat)

Egg whites

I love eggs. I know many people do. I recommend them all the
time as a great source of protein. But eggs, especially the whites,
can aggravate existing autoimmune problems. The egg white
exists as a means to protect the yolk (a growing life form) from any
microbial attacks. It does this by way of a specific enzyme called
lysozyme (there are a few other enzymes involved, but lysozyme
is the one that aggravates autoimmunity the most). Lysozyme
is a strong substance that is meant to help break apart cellular
membranes. Inasmuch as it is hard to digest, this can exacerbate
inflammation and autoimmunity. Moreover, egg whites can
permeate the lining of an already leaky gut and possibly cause the
immune system to react.[12] So for now, you are going to enjoy only
egg yolks. You can reintroduce the whole egg after a few weeks on
the *Body Belief* eating plan.

Alcohol and coffee

These two beverages are a favorite to many, but the truth is they're not the best for our health. Alcohol is a known toxic agent that causes an increase in intestinal permeability. In excess (more than five drinks a week), it's really not good for you, but I'd be lying if I told you I didn't enjoy some alcohol here and there.

When it comes to alcohol, the most important thing to do before drinking is to reconnect to yourself and know why you are drinking. Are you drinking out of joy or out of stress? If it's for joy, then go for it *in moderation*. If it's because you're stressed or sad or you want to numb out, then go back to Chapter 4 and use your tools to work through those emotions.

You will get to a point where you can try these drinks again, but coffee must always be organic (because nonorganic coffee contains a very high pesticide load that is very harmful to your health), and alcohol should be in the form of highly distilled spirits like vodka or tequila, which are the easiest for your body to process, free of added sugar, and, due to the distillation process, gluten-free. But for the purposes of maximizing your health and vitality, I am going to have you eliminate them—*except for the occasional cup, say once a week, of organic coffee*—for the first six weeks of the *Body Belief* eating plan. After that, you can enjoy a cup of organic black or green tea three to five times per week, if you still feel healthy while doing it.

Now we get to talk about *all* the delicious and nutritious foods you *can* eat!

The *Body Belief* Foods

I know that by now you are wondering, "What can I eat on this plan?" In truth, there's a lot you can eat in the form of protein, fat, veggies, and fruit. Think wild Alaskan salmon with preserved lemon and cauliflower rice (and it actually has the texture of rice), or homemade meatballs served over a bed of spaghetti squash noodles with delicious "no-mato" sauce (a nightshade-free version of marinara sauce), or baked cod with braised kale. There are tender pork chops with homemade sauerkraut and sautéed spinach, or a fresh, juicy apple in a cinnamon-coconut-milk smoothie, or a sweet potato topped with ghee, or warming ginger bone broth with diced avocado. Or perhaps try a cozy butternut squash soup with chunks of grilled chicken, or homemade coconut yogurt with fresh berries. There's so much you can eat on this new plan!

Without further ado, I am going to share with you all the nutrient-dense and body-loving foods you can enjoy on your new eating plan. But first, three caveats:

1. Assume that everything on this list is organic, and that all animal products are pasture-raised, free-range, grass-fed, and hormone- and antibiotic-free. Getting locally grown and in-season food are major pluses.

2. This diet is carnivorous, so please don't be afraid of animal protein. These foods are rich in essential nutrients like iron, B vitamins, and saturated fats, which make them great for reducing inflammation, regulating your immune system, healing your leaky gut, and radically improving your health. A serving of meat or fish is about three to four ounces, or the surface area of your palm.

3. Fat is your friend. Don't be afraid of saturated fats; they are loaded with fat-soluble vitamins like A, K, and D that are essential to your healing. Saturated fats found in animal protein keep your blood sugar even and your energy high, and they will not give you high cholesterol.

What if I'm a vegan or a vegetarian?

I'll be the first to admit, this diet isn't very vegetarian- or vegan-friendly. That's not because I don't respect your decision not to eat animal products, but because animal products are the most nutrient-dense and healing foods that exist. If there is any room for flexibility in your diet, I am hoping you can find a way to eat at least egg yolks, cultured ghee, fish, fish stock, and even some collagen protein.

OK, here are all the foods that are going to help you radically shift your health and heal autoimmunity:

Homemade Bone Broth: Homemade bone broths are rich in calcium, magnesium, phosphorus, glucosamine, and chondroitin, all of which are necessary for a properly functioning immune system. Most importantly, bone broths are rich in gelatin. Gelatin is a phenomenal source of protein that provides our bodies with the essence they need to engender health, longevity, and vitality; and it is necessary for healing leaky gut and intestinal permeability. Bone broth is the key to healing from autoimmunity. The PURIFY phase of the *Body Belief* eating plan includes a lot of bone broth; but for now, understand that bone broth will be a big part of your new way of eating. My goal is for you to consume six to eight ounces of bone broth daily. Sip it like a tea, add it to your favorite foods, or cook with it—just get it in. If consuming that much bone broth doesn't feel good to you, you can substitute two scoops per day of a gelatin supplement; Vital Proteins Beef Gelatin and Collagen Peptides, and Dr. Axe's Bone Broth Protein, are great choices. But keep in mind that it is ideal that you substitute the powder for broth no more than half the time (or three days/week).

If your body is not used to eating bone broth, you may have to gradually work up to six to eight ounces daily. The key here is to listen to your body. If you feel any discomfort or digestive symptoms, back off the broth and cut my recommendations in half. After 10 to 14 days, try to increase your intake and note how you feel.

Egg yolk: Eat 1-2 per day. We will add egg whites toward the end of the *Body Belief* eating plan, but for now you can still enjoy the yolks from pasture-fed organic eggs, consuming 8 to 12 per week. Egg yolks from pastured hens are deeply nutrient-dense—rich in fertility-boosting omega-3 fatty acids, vitamins A and E, and choline. Make sure the eggs you buy are from chickens that were never fed soy, because the soy proteins from the feed can get into the eggs, which will then cause an autoimmune reaction. (The eggs should be pastured or free-range; if they are "vegetarian fed," that means they were fed soy.) To ensure you aren't exposed to any egg whites, after separating the yolk from the white you should rinse the yolk to get 100 percent of the egg white off before eating.

Some great ways to add the yolks to your daily diet are to stir them into your daily broth for a delicious egg drop soup; to bake the yolk inside a halved and pitted avocado (yes! It's called a "yolkocado" and it's amazing); to use the yolk as the binder for meatballs or meatloaf; or to make eggnog or mayonnaise. You can also just pan fry the yolk in coconut oil or ghee for a quick bite to eat.

Meat and Poultry: Eat 6 to 10 servings per week of grass-fed, hormone-free, and antibiotic-free meat, such as lamb, venison, grass-fed beef, buffalo, pork, chicken, bison, or turkey. Bacon and sausage are allowed one to two times a week total, as long as they are nitrate- and gluten-free, and contain no artificial sweeteners or spices beyond those that are allowed (see p. 99). Grass-fed beef is the only beef you should eat; and pastured, free-range poultry is the only poultry you should eat. Pan sear, grill, or broil the meat in a healthy fat, some broth, or both.

Your Water

I know we are talking about all of the *Body Belief* foods, but I also need to address something very important for you: water. Not just your intake, but the quality of water you are drinking.

Intake: Generally, I recommend that water be your primary beverage, that you drink it at room temperature, and that you consume about half your body weight in ounces each day. But if that feels like too much or too little water to you, rely on your body's built-in water radar: thirst. If you are thirsty, drink. If you are not, don't force yourself.

Quality: The truth is, nearly all the water available to you is of poor quality and filled with run-off that contains many of the chemicals I want you to avoid. My advice is to invest in a high-quality water filter and install it in your home. Personally, I use the Berkey system with the black filters at home, but there are a few other great ones to choose from. (The Environmental Working Group [EWG] put out a great guide at www.ewg.org/tap-water/getawaterfilter.php. I have more information on this topic for you on my website at AimeeRaupp.com/BodyBelief.) I also feel it is best to avoid bottled water, especially in plastic bottles. Your best bet is to buy a stainless steel or glass water bottle and fill it up with your filtered water at home before you go out.

Liver: Yes, liver as in the organ meat. Eat one 3- to 4-ounce serving per week of liver from small fish or pastured/grass-fed animals (cod, chicken, and lamb are the best sources). Liver is one of the best antioxidant, anti-autoimmune, nutrient-dense foods that exists. It is a rich source of folate, vitamin B12, pantothenic acid, riboflavin, inositol, niacin, selenium, and vitamin A. A single 3.5 ounce portion of pan-fried chicken livers contains three times as much folate as an equivalent serving of raw spinach.

If the idea of eating liver makes your stomach turn, you can take it in pill form; my favorite sources are DrRons.com and Vital Proteins. Both companies make liver pills from grass-fed cattle. Take two pills per day to meet the recommended intake. *If you are taking a blood-thinning medication, consult with your doctor before taking liver pills.*

Seafood: Eat 8 to 12 servings per week of seafood, which can include deep-sea coldwater fish, wild-caught seafood, and shellfish. You can eat any of these: salmon, sardines, halibut, snapper, trout, herring, sardines, tilapia, mackerel, anchovies, catfish, mahi mahi, mussels, octopus, prawns, scallops, crab, shrimp, squid, oysters, clams, and cod. They are rich in omega-3 fatty acids such as DHA and EPA, vitamins D and B12, and zinc. Broil, steam, or grill the seafood using a healthy fat. You can find other great options in your particular region of the country at Monterey Bay Aquarium's Seafood Watch (www.seafoodwatch.org).

Fish Roe: Eat 1 ounce one to two times per week, as fish roe has a high ratio of omega-3 to omega-6 fatty acids. Our goal is to decrease omega-6 fatty acids and increase omega-3 fatty acids, in order to lower systemic inflammation in your body. Fish roe goes by a few names: caviar, *tobiko* (flying fish roe), and *ikura* (salmon roe). I prefer tobiko, because the eggs are tiny and don't taste too fishy.

Cultured Ghee: Eat 1 tablespoon per day. The key here is that the ghee be cultured or fermented. Ghee is technically a dairy product, but in the process of making it the milk proteins are not entirely removed, so it can have trace amounts of casein and/ or lactose. So if someone has a dairy allergy, ghee still isn't safe for them, since there's no guarantee that it's dairy-free. However, when ghee is cultured it goes through a process whereby fermentable bacteria eat up any remaining milk proteins. One product in particular, Pure Indian Foods Grass-Fed & Organic Cultured Ghee, even sends their ghee off for lab testing to ensure it's free of all dairy proteins. With that, I recommend you get this brand and this brand only. (By the time this book is published or you get your hands on it, there may be other brands out there that are fermenting or culturing their ghee and ensuring it's dairy free, so read the label and ask a lot of questions and buy only ghee that is cultured or fermented and guaranteed to be free of dairy proteins.) *Or* you can quite easily make it at home. Ghee is a superbly nutrient-dense food and a potent source of fat-soluble vitamins A and K2, both of which positively influence health and immunity. Cook with it, add it to your broth, and slab it on your veggies.

Organic Oils and Fats: Consume 1 to 2 tablespoons per day of organic oils and fats, such as extra virgin olive oil, avocado oil, coconut oil, palm oil, lard, tallow, and ghee (which got its own section because it's *that* good for you). They are rich in essential fatty acids that will help regulate your immune system and heal leaky gut. All of the oils should be organic and cold-pressed; all of the fats should be from grass-fed sources. Avoid all other oils and fats. Cook with them or put them on your salads.

Healthy Fats You Should Cook With

Healthy fats play a critical role in your body—they enhance nutrient absorption, boost immune function, help your body make essential fatty acids, and provide a rich source of fat-soluble vitamins, all of which are imperative to restoring your health and your body's capacity to heal itself. Healthy fat is *not* margarine, canola oil, or any refined and chemically extracted vegetable oil (like corn or soy). These substances are processed and far from healthy, so steer clear of them!

Any time I mention cooking with a healthy fat, I am talking about one of the following:

Coconut oil (extra virgin, raw, and cold-pressed)

Cultured ghee (from grass-fed/pastured cows)

Lard (from grass-fed/pastured pork)

Tallow (from grass-fed/pastured beef)

The other oils I mention in this section are not for cooking, but rather are for making dressings or marinades. Do not use them to cook!

Vegetables: You should have one serving of vegetables with each meal at minimum, with a total of three to five servings per day! A serving size for vegetables is ½ cup or 4 ounces. Eat a variety of colors and types of vegetables each day, *except* for the nightshades (p. 8). Prepare by steaming, sautéing, or roasting them in one of my recommended healthy fats. You can also blanch some veggies like spinach or kale and add them to a smoothie. Once or twice a week you can also make a fresh vegetable juice and drink your veggies, keeping in mind my advice about cooked vs. raw foods (p. 100).

When you cook your vegetables, be sure you make them al dente, which means "to the tooth," or slightly undercooked; over-cooked vegetables lose most of their nutrients.

Eat loads of:

- Leafy greens: lettuce, spinach, kale, chard, collards, dandelion greens, cilantro, parsley, endive, napa cabbage, watercress, and kelp

- Cruciferous veggies: arugula, radishes, radicchio, turnips, mustard greens, broccoli, brussels sprouts, cabbage, cauliflower, and bok choy

- Onions, scallions, garlic, leeks, shallots, spring onions, and chives

- Root veggies: carrots, beets, jicama, squash, pumpkin, rutabaga, turnips, and parsnip

- Sweet potatoes and yams

- Sea vegetables: arame, dulse, kombu, nori, and wakame

- Other veggies: artichokes, capers, celery, cucumber, zucchini, olives, and okra

Prebiotic-rich foods: eat one serving a day. Prebiotics are foods that deliver digestible fibers, and they help to restore healthy gut bacteria and to heal intestinal permeability. Eat foods like Jerusalem artichoke, dandelion greens, chicory roots, cabbage, garlic, onion, leeks, asparagus, banana, apple, jicama, and any sea vegetable. Most of these foods are mentioned in other categories in the *Body Belief* eating plan, but I want to point them out since they are great specifically for helping improve your digestion and heal leaky gut.

Note: Prebiotics are not to be confused with probiotics (p. 114).

Fermented foods: eat 2 tablespoons of foods like sauerkraut, kimchi, pickled ginger, or one 4- to 6-ounce serving per day of water kefir, coconut-milk kefir, coconut-milk yogurt, and kombucha. These foods supply your digestive system with good bacteria that are essential to regulating your immune system, healing any intestinal permeability, breaking down the food you eat, and assimilating the nutrients from that food.

> *If you are finding that the prebiotic and/or fermented foods I recommend are giving you digestive discomfort, cut my recommended intake of these foods in half until your body begins to tolerate them better. These types of foods are highly healing to the lining of the gut, but if there is leaky gut, sometimes the body can't tolerate these foods right away.*

Fruit: Fruits are a great source of vitamins, minerals, fiber, and antioxidants, though they are typically high in sugar. Any food with a high sugar content, even if it's natural sugar, needs to be eaten in moderation. Eating too much sugar can cause insulin resistance and create inflammation in your body. I want you to indulge mainly in fruits with the lowest amount of sugar, and then once in a while have some really sweet fruit. Of course, it's ideal to eat fruits that are in season for your region.

Eat six to eight servings per week of a low-sugared fruit: melons, berries, grapefruit, and avocado. Yes, that's any melon and any berry.

Eat only two to four servings per week of moderate-to-high-sugared fruits: apples, apricots, kiwi, nectarine, papaya, plum, pomegranate, pears, plum, peach, citrus (all others except grapefruit), banana, mango, pineapple, plantains, watermelon, dates, and fresh figs.

Dried fruits and 100 percent pure juices, NOT from concentrate: Both of these are very high in sugar and should be consumed very sparingly—they are not recommended in the first six weeks of the *Body Belief* eating plan, and after that should be consumed no more than once every two weeks.

Spices and Seasonings

There is a lot of cooking with your new way of eating, so I want to let you know all the spices and seasonings (dried or fresh) you can use in this plan. If you don't see a spice or seasoning on this list, that means you can't use it until you are at least four weeks into the REAWAKEN phase of the *Body Belief* eating plan. Here are the spices you can use:

Balm (lemon balm)	Basil leaves (sweet)
Bay leaves (laurel leaves)	Chamomile
Chervil	Chives
Cilantro (coriander Leaf)	Cinnamon/cassia
Cloves	Dill weed
Garlic	Ginger
Horseradish	Lavender
Mace	Marjoram leaves
Onion powder	Oregano leaves
Parsley	Peppermint
Rosemary	Saffron
Sage	Salt
Savory leaves	Spearmint
Tarragon	Thyme
Turmeric	

Use in moderation (one to two times per week) while in the first four weeks of the REAWAKEN phase:

Allspice	Caraway
Cardamom	Juniper
Black pepper	White pepper
Green peppercorns	Pink peppercorns
Star anise	Vanilla bean

Eat more cooked food than raw food. By raw, I mean foods that are cold or uncooked. This is a very important piece of the *Body Belief* eating plan, because eating too many raw foods can hamper digestion and create more inflammation in your body. Plus, from a TOM perspective, cold or raw foods are harder to digest and are therefore hard to get healthy, abundant, and vital qi from. So when following this plan, be sure that you are eating most of your foods cooked. That doesn't mean you can't have a vegetable juice now and again; just have it in moderation. So as your body heals, you can indulge in more raw foods; but for now I want you to be eating 80 to 85 percent of your foods cooked.

Chapter Eight

The *Body Belief* Eating
Plan: Step by Step

The PREP Phase

The PREP phase can last anywhere from a few days to a few weeks, but I do want it to end at some point so you can move into the next phase of this plan. In the prep phase you are going to prep mentally, emotionally, physically, and nutritionally for your new way of eating and living. Just as you are finding the time to use the tools from Chapters 4 and 5, I want you to begin to see how this new lifestyle is going to fit into your life. What changes do you need to make? Do you need to go food shopping more regularly? Do you need to shift your morning routine to allow time for cooking, or can you find time over the weekend to cook and prepare food for the week? Do you need to start reading labels to see what it is you're actually eating on a regular basis? Do you need a few days to wrap your head around all of what I am recommending? Wherever you are, it's exactly where you're meant to be. And know this: I have taken many steps to make this as easy as possible for you (for instance, I have created a sample seven-day REAWAKEN menu plan for you that you can find on p. 112, so that you can really make this happen). So trust that you are supported. Move forward with this *Body Belief* eating plan from a place of kindness and compassion for yourself.

Here's what I want you to focus on in this PREP phase:

1. Begin eliminating from your diet the food*stuffs* you are never to eat again. They are: gluten, soy, added sugar, artificial sweeteners, food chemicals, and processed vegetable oils (p. 83). If you're already living this way, skip to number two. If this is all brand new to you, spend at least seven days in this phase to start wrapping your head around the idea that you're going to eat way fewer, if any, processed and packaged foods ever again, and a lot less bread, pasta, diet soda, fat-free anything, crackers, cookies, donuts, pretzels, pancakes, and muffins. Take comfort, though: later, you can enjoy some yummy gluten-free pancakes and muffins, and there are some great gluten-free pastas you can have *in moderation* when you reintroduce grains. Also, be sure to check *all* your supplements and vitamins for any of these food*stuffs*, as they can hide out in them. If you discover that any of your vitamins or supplements contain food*stuffs*, stop them immediately. I will have you introduce new supplements once you enter the REAWAKEN phase of this plan.

2. Start food shopping for organic, fresh (local and in season if possible) vegetables and fruit, along with high-quality meats, fish, and fat. Be sure to skip buying *any* nightshade vegetables. Make a list of 10 to 20 items so that you have a variety of vegetables, fruits, and proteins, which is very important. However, don't go crazy with buying a ton of perishable fruits and veggies if you're not starting the REAWAKEN phase within a few days.

3. Start cutting back or completely removing alcohol, coffee, grains, dairy, and beans from your diet. Do this at your own pace. Even if you limit your intake of grains (gluten-free only) to just once a day, three

times a week, that's a great place to start. The same goes for dairy: either cut it out straightaway or begin limiting it to one serving three times a week (organic and full-fat dairy only). As for coffee, either cut it out completely or cut your usual daily intake in half and make sure the coffee you are drinking is organic. The same goes for alcohol. It's ideal to cut it out entirely, but if you'd rather ease into it, then cut back to three, or at the very most five, drinks a week. And if you can, cut beans out altogether starting now; at the very least, limit them to one serving once or twice per week.

4. Make your first batch of bone broth. Choose from one of my recipes (pp. 180–187) and dive in. It's really quite easy to make broth, especially if you have a crockpot or an Instant Pot. If this is all brand-new for you, consider investing in a crockpot or Instant Pot to simplify the broth-making process. The next two phases of this plan, PURIFY and REAWAKEN, require a lot of broth—about 60 ounces per week—so get started with this as soon as you can. Don't fret: in the recipes, I go over not just how to cook the broths but how to store and freeze them as well, so you have plenty to last you.

5. Take 5 to 10 minutes each day and visualize a healthier version of you. You can make this visualization practice your meditation for the days/weeks of your PREP phase. Here's what I want you to do: Sit or lie comfortably, close your eyes, and begin to see a healthier version of yourself. See yourself living and owning this *Body Belief* eating plan. See yourself cooking and food shopping. See yourself feeling the best you have felt in years, and enjoying your food. See yourself feeling proud and excited about your new lifestyle—really get into how it would look in your current life. After you spend time

doing the visualization, take two to three minutes to journal about all that you felt and saw. If any resistance or negative beliefs come up, go back to Chapter 5 and work through them. Keep up this practice for as long as you need. See yourself doing this, see your health thriving, see yourself feeling your best. You deserve it.

OK, that wraps up the PREP phase. As I said, take as much time as you need in this phase—three days or three weeks or even three months. Whatever works for you. Remember, there are hundreds of others going through this with you, so reach out and share how you're feeling, because support is key to making this lifestyle shift.

The PURIFY Phase

The PURIFY phase is going to jump-start your body and its cells, and set the stage for radical healing. It is meant to last 11 days, consisting of 4 days during which you are eating a mix of specific foods, fat, and broth; followed by 3 days of all broth with some fat and veggies; and then another 4 days of specific foods, fat, and broth. Eating this way for 11 days will help reduce inflammation in your body and get you into the *Body Belief* eating plan mind-set. Truth: During the first couple of days in the PURIFY phase, you may not feel great. You may even feel worse than you currently do. But stay the course, because I assure that you are going to start feeling really good by day 5 or 6, and it is *so* worth it. When you are about to start the PURIFY phase, get yourself a journal so you can keep notes about how you feel on a daily basis. I want you to keep this journal throughout both the PURIFY and REAWAKEN phases, writing about how you feel going through each phase and how you feel after each phase. What changes do you notice in your red-flag symptoms, your digestion, your energy levels, your mood, your sleep? Do you feel accomplished after finishing it? Do you feel supported while you are in the midst of following this program? What beliefs come up for you while you are doing it, and do they shift from being negative to more positive? Noting all of this is going to help you as you move into your state of reawakened health.

Please note: in the PURIFY phase there is no fruit, vitamins, or supplements (your body can use a break from any supplements for the time being); consume only the foods and recipes mentioned below. And don't skip the Epsom-salt baths, as they are a big part of the cleansing process. Here are the specifics:

Days 1 through 4:

- Wake up. Take a few minutes to meditate, visualize, and breathe deeply. Take a few more minutes to journal about three things you appreciate about your body. Also write down three physical symptoms you hope to see improvement in during the PURIFY phase.

- Make yourself a mug of fresh ginger tea with the juice from half a lemon squeezed into it (see recipe on p. 197), *or* a mug of hot water with a shot of apple cider vinegar or juice from half a lemon squeezed into it. If you really need some caffeine, choose between organic black tea and organic green tea (no sugar, no cream) and add the juice from half a lemon. (The properties from the lemon juice and the apple cider vinegar are very important here, and aid in your digestion and healing process, so make sure not to skip that part).

- Prepare your breakfast: Bone Broth Egg Drop Soup (p. 176) *or* Coconut-Milk Yogurt (p. 174) *or* Golden Turmeric Sipping Broth (p. 177) *or* the Purify Smoothie (p. 197). Be sure to eat it within 30 minutes of waking up.

- Two to three hours after breakfast, snack on 6 to 8 ounces of kombucha *or* coconut kefir and a sweet potato with a healthy fat, *or* a cup of Yummy Butternut Squash Soup (p. 177), *or* a yolkocado (p. 188), *or* the Purify Smoothie (p. 197).

- At some point during your day, have 6 to 8 ounces of Liver Support Juice (p. 196). And throughout your day be sure to drink filtered water to the point of feeling hydrated and satiated.

- Two to three hours later, have lunch: your choice of grilled protein and sautéed veggies cooked in a healthy fat. For your protein, choose wild salmon *or* cod *or* grass-fed beef *or* lamb. For your veggies, choose spinach, kale, broccoli, asparagus, cauliflower, or beets. Use only parsley, ginger, turmeric, cinnamon, cilantro, or pink Himalayan sea salt to season your food. *To make it easier on yourself, prepare two servings of this meal and have one for lunch and the other for dinner.*

- Two to three hours after lunch, snack on a half cup of sauerkraut and a sweet potato with a healthy fat, *or* a cup of Yummy Butternut Squash Soup (p. 177) or a yolkocado (p. 188).

- Two to three hours later, have dinner: your choice of grilled protein and sautéed veggies cooked in a healthy fat. The options are the same as they were for lunch. For your protein, choose wild salmon *or* cod *or* grass-fed beef *or* lamb. For your veggies, choose spinach, kale, broccoli, asparagus, cauliflower, or beets. Use only parsley, ginger, turmeric, cinnamon, cilantro, or pink Himalayan sea salt to season your food.

- Two hours later have 4 ounces of bone broth.

- At some point during your day, soak for 10 to 20 minutes in a warm bath with 2 cups of Epsom salts *or* magnesium chloride flakes. Meditate or practice visualization during your tub soak.

- Twenty minutes before falling asleep, spray the soles of your feet with magnesium oil (six squirts per foot). See recipe on p. 199.

- Find a few minutes before bed to do one of the exercises from Chapter 5, and keep on that path of renewing your beliefs. Your healing depends on it!

> ## Epsom *or* Magnesium Chloride salt baths
>
> Soaking in a tub of hot water with a cup or two of Epsom (a.k.a. magnesium sulfate) *or* magnesium chloride salts can be highly therapeutic, not only in this cleanse phase but throughout your healing process. Taking a bath with either of these salts has an anti-inflammatory effect on the body, and has been proven to be an effective pain reliever and stress reducer. Indulge and let yourself soak in a warm tub with some of these salts as often as you can! You won't regret it.

Days 5 through 7:

- For the next three days of the PURIFY phase, you are going to consume more broth than anything else. This is what is going to heal your gut and boost your blood, qi, and essence, which will truly begin to reawaken your vitality. It may be challenging, but stay the course, as your body will feel so good as a result of this part of the PURIFY phase.

- Wake up. Take a few minutes to meditate, visualize, and breathe deeply. Take a few more minutes to journal about three things you appreciate about your health. Write down three physical symptoms that have improved since beginning this new lifestyle. Even if they aren't dramatic improvements just yet, note some positive changes you see in these symptoms.

- Make yourself a mug of ginger tea with the juice from half a lemon squeezed into it. There is no caffeine for these three days.

- Prepare your breakfast, either: Bone Broth Egg Drop Soup (p. 176) *or* Coconut-Milk Yogurt (p. 174) *or* Golden Turmeric Sipping Broth (p. 177) *or* the Purify Smoothie (p. 197). Be sure to eat within 30 minutes of waking up.

- Two to three hours after breakfast, snack on 6 to 8 ounces of water or coconut kefir and a sweet potato with a healthy fat, *or* a cup of Yummy Butternut Squash soup (p. 177), *or* a yolkocado (p. 188).

- Two to three hours later and for the rest of the day, using your hunger as a cue for when to eat (but try your best to eat every two to three hours), have the following: 8 ounces of Turmeric Ginger Bone Broth (p. 187) *or* Bone Broth Egg Drop Soup (p. 176) *or* Golden Turmeric Sipping Broth (p. 177) *or* Yummy Butternut Squash soup (p. 177) *or* the Purify Smoothie (p. 197). If you are feeling hungry and need more food, you can add half an avocado to your meals, or half a sweet potato with a healthy fat (limit yourself to a maximum of one full avocado, two sweet potatoes, and two egg yolks per day).

- At some point during your day, have 6 to 8 ounces of Liver Support Juice (p. 196). And throughout your day be sure to drink filtered water to the point of feeling hydrated and satiated.

- At some point during your day, soak for 10 to 20 minutes in a warm bath with 2 cups of Epsom salts.

- Twenty minutes before falling asleep, spray the soles of your feet with magnesium oil (six squirts per foot). See recipe on p. 199.

- Find a few minutes before bed to do one of the exercises from Chapter 5, and keep on that path of renewing your beliefs.

Exercise during the Purify phase: It is recommended to do moderate exercise five days per week for 30 to 45 minutes. The ideal exercises are yoga, Pilates, core workouts, mini trampoline-jumping, cycling, walking, or elliptical. Do not exercise to the point of feeling exhausted; exercise to feel invigorated and energized. If you are feeling fatigued from exercise, cut back to three days per week for 30 minutes at a time.

Days 8 through 11:

- The last four days of the PURIFY phase are the same as the first four days; here you will begin reintroducing more food after three days of mainly consuming broth.

- Wake up. Take a few minutes to meditate, visualize, and breathe deeply. Take a few more minutes to journal about three things you appreciate about yourself, and about the commitment you have made to the *Body Belief* eating plan. Write down three physical symptoms that have improved since beginning this new lifestyle.

- Make yourself a mug of ginger tea with the juice from half a lemon squeezed into it. If you really need some caffeine, choose between organic black tea or organic green tea (no sugar, no cream), and add the juice from half a lemon.

- Prepare your breakfast: either Bone Broth Egg Drop Soup (p. 176) *or* Coconut-Milk Yogurt (p. 174) *or* Golden Turmeric Sipping Broth (p. 177) *or* the Purify Smoothie (p. 197). Be sure to eat within 30 minutes of waking up.

- Two to three hours after breakfast, snack on 6 to 8 ounces of water or coconut kefir and a sweet potato with a healthy fat, *or* a cup of Yummy Butternut

Squash Soup (p. 177), *or* a yolkocado (p. 188), *or* the Purify Smoothie (p. 197).

- At some point during your day, have 6 to 8 ounces of Liver Support Juice (p. 196). And throughout your day be sure to drink filtered water to the point of feeling hydrated and satiated.

- Two to three hours later, have lunch: your choice of grilled protein or sautéed veggies cooked in a healthy fat. For your protein, choose from wild salmon, cod, grass-fed beef, or lamb. For your veggies, choose spinach, kale, broccoli, asparagus, cauliflower, asparagus, or beets. Use only parsley, ginger, turmeric, cinnamon, cilantro, or pink Himalayan sea salt to season your food. *To make it easier on yourself, prepare two servings of this meal and have one for lunch and the other for dinner.*

- Two to three hours after lunch, snack on a half cup of sauerkraut and a sweet potato with cultured ghee, *or* a cup of Yummy Butternut Squash Soup (p. 177), *or* a yolkocado (p. 188), *or* the Purify Smoothie (p. 197).

- Two to three hours later, have dinner: grilled protein and sautéed veggies cooked in a healthy fat. For your protein, you can choose wild salmon, cod, grass-fed beef, or lamb; for your veggies, you can choose spinach, kale, broccoli, asparagus, cauliflower, or beets. Use only parsley, ginger, turmeric, cinnamon, cilantro, and pink Himalayan sea salt to season your food.

- Two hours later, have 4 ounces of bone broth.

- At some point during your day, soak for 10 to 20 minutes in a warm bath with 2 cups of Epsom salts.

- Twenty minutes before falling asleep, spray the soles of your feet with magnesium oil (six squirts per foot). See recipe on p. 199.

- Find a few minutes before bed to do one of the exercises from Chapter 5, and keep on that path of renewing your beliefs.

Unlike other diets, detoxes, or cleanses, this PURIFY phase will not leave you starving and irritable. Rather, this way of eating is filled with nutrient-dense and satisfying broths, soups, and tasty side dishes that are going to reboot your body, boost your qi, and begin to repair your leaky gut. You can always revisit this phase or do it for longer if you feel your body needs it, but try following my advice exactly at first.

The REAWAKEN Phase

After you make it through the PURIFY phase you are going to feel enlivened, lighter, and clearer. You may even have lost a few pounds. On the first few days of the REAWAKEN phase, revisit your journal entries over the last 11 days to remind yourself of the changes you are seeing in your body and the shifts in how you are feeling. The daily journaling is even more important in this phase because you need to be reconnected to you so you can be tuned in and notice how your body feels when you reintroduce certain foods.

Now that you have reduced your inflammation, taken the toxic load off of your body, and cleansed from the damage done to your cells, you are ready to REAWAKEN. In this phase, the focus is on healing your autoimmunity and maintaining the health of your cells so your body can thrive. For the first three weeks of this phase you will be able to eat any and all of the *Body Belief* foods— lots of broth, protein, vegetables, fat, and fruit; you can even have some caffeine again. After that, each subsequent week you can reintroduce a food group from the foods that don't support your autoimmunity section (on p. 84), and see how your body feels and how it reacts (or doesn't) to the new food. Of course, reintroduce only the foods that you would like to. You can maintain the diet you had in the PURIFY phase for as long as you like, but reintroduce only certain foods, or reintroduce all the foods that I list in the REAWAKEN phase. Regardless of whether you reintroduce only some or all the foods in the plan, there is a specific order in which to reintroduce the foods, so as to manage what could potentially react with your immune system and aggravate auto-immunity. So please follow this phase step by step, and really pay attention to your body, its red-flag symptoms, and any digestive issues that come up.

Weeks One, Two, and Three

You can eat any of the *Body Belief* foods (p. 90) while making sure you stick to the following rules:

- Consume 6 to 8 ounces of broth each day (or have a smoothie with the collagen peptides and bone broth powder; 1 scoop of each)

- Eat no more than 1 to 2 egg yolks per day (having egg yolks isn't mandatory)

- Eat a serving of protein (about 3 to 4 ounces, or the size of your palm) with every meal. It's ideal to consume 6 to 10 servings of meat each week and 8 to 12 servings of seafood.

- Eat breakfast within the first 30 minutes of waking, and be sure to eat every two to three hours thereafter.

- Get in 3 to 5 servings of a variety of vegetables each day. Think about eating all the colors of the rainbow.

- Eat some fruit (p. 98).

- Allow yourself a maximum of 1 cup of organic black tea or green tea daily.

- Eat more cooked food than raw. Cook all foods in healthy fats, making sure to consume at least 1 tablespoon of cultured ghee daily and 1 to 2 tablespoons of the other healthy fats daily.

- Get in one serving each day of a fermented food.

- Get in one serving each day of a prebiotic food.

- Get in 6 to 8 ounces of the Liver Support Juice (p. 196) four times per week.

- Drink plenty of room-temperature filtered water, to the point of feeling your thirst quenched.

- Do moderate exercise five days per week for 30 to 45 minutes at a time (ideal exercise: yoga, Pilates, core workouts, mini trampoline-jumping, cycling, walking, or elliptical). *Do not exercise to the point of feeling exhausted; exercise to feel invigorated and energized. If you are feeling fatigued from exercise, cut back to three days per week for 30 minutes at a time.*

- Once a week, get in 3 to 4 ounces of organ meat, such as liver (which can also be taken in capsule form).

- Once or twice a week, get in 1 ounce (½ teaspoon) of fish roe.

- At some point during your day, soak for 10 to 20 minutes in a warm bath with 2 cups of Epsom salts.

- Take only the supplements I recommend (p. 114).

- Spray the soles of your feet 20 minutes before bed each night with magnesium oil (ideally six sprays per foot; see recipe on p. 199).

- Be sure to meditate, journal, or practice visualization every day. Revisit the tools from Chapters 4 and 5 and weave them into your daily life. Take time before each meal to practice what I call "Food Gratitude," where you thank your food for nourishing your body and helping you heal (examples of Food Gratitude statements are on p. x).

- Sleep seven to eight hours each night.

Supplements and Vitamins: What to Take to Help Your Body Heal and Thrive

During the PURIFY phase of the *Body Belief* eating plan, I recommended that you stop taking all of your supplements and vitamins. Now it is time to add them back in. However, I want you to add only the ones I recommend as your body is going through a healing process and we need to support that process, not inundate it with too many vitamins and supplements. Rest assured, the vitamin/supplement regimen below, in conjunction with all the amazing foods you are eating, will give your body all that it needs to heal and thrive. When you are three months into the *Body Belief* program *and* your red-flag symptoms are about 85 to 90 percent improved, then (and only then) you can add more vitamins/supplements. But keep in mind that your new diet and way of life are giving your body most of what it needs. The supplements I recommend you take to further optimize your healing are:

- **Spirulina:** Spirulina is a freshwater blue-green algae that's nearly 3.5 *billion* years old. It's a tremendously rich source of protein, essential fatty acids, and vitamins like B_1, B_2, B_3, B_6, B_9, C, D, and E. Bottom line: Spirulina is full of immune-enhancing anti-oxidants perfect for helping you heal from autoimmunity. Spirulina comes in tablet, capsule, or powder form. Whichever brand you decide to get, take it as directed on the bottle. My all-time favorite, top-notch brands of spirulina are:

    Nutrex Pure Hawaiian Organic Spirulina (take as directed)
    Garden of Life Perfect Food (take as directed)
    Pure Synergy Superfoods (take as directed)

    Spirulina is one of those supplements that can be taken long term, because it is a food. I consider it nature's multivitamin; hence I recommend taking a dose of spirulina daily for the rest of your life.

- **Probiotics:** The word probiotic means "for life." Probiotics are the good bacteria found in your digestive tract. Taking a probiotic supplement helps to maintain the natural balance of good and bad bacteria in your body, improves your digestion, and boosts your immune system. I'm sure you've heard of probiotics before—they're often touted as natural components of certain mainstream foods like Dannon's Activa yogurt. Like all nutritional supplements, probiotics come in different shapes and sizes, and some forms are not worth your time or money. The key thing about ingesting a probiotic is that it needs to survive the harsh acidity in your stomach and make it to your small intestine so that it can actually give you some of its benefits. The *Body Belief* eating plan is having you eat plenty of foods with naturally occurring probiotic activity, as the goal is to heal your gut. That said, I want you to take the following probiotic supplements as I direct:

Begin with taking Prescript-Assist (start off with a capsule a day for four weeks and then go to two capsules per day); continue taking two capsules per day of Prescript-Assist until most of your red-flag symptoms subside or are at least 85 to 90 percent better. At that point you can switch to another probiotic. I recommend MegaFood's MegaFlora Plus 50 billion; take one per day and continue for at least six months.

Once you are feeling mostly healed, as long as you're eating probiotic rich foods, you don't need a daily probiotic; taking one a few times each week is just fine.

- **Digestive enzymes:** Taking these will help ensure that the foods you are eating are fully digested, decreasing the chance that partially digested foods particles and proteins are damaging your intestines and worsening leaky gut. I recommend the following products (take as directed):

  Pure Digestive Enzymes Ultra
  Dr. Axe organic enzymes
  Wobenzym N

  Just as with probiotics, once you are seeing major improvements in your state of health and in your red-flag symptoms, you don't need to be taking digestive enzymes on a regular basis. In fact, if you take them for too long, too regularly, your body will become dependent upon them for digesting food. So take these during your first three months of your Body Belief protocol, and as you are feeling better, cut back and let your body do the job of digesting its food all on its own.

- **L-Glutamine:** This amino acid is critical for healing leaky gut. Glutamine powder is an essential amino acid supplement and a powerful antioxidant. It helps regulate immune function, has anti-inflammatory actions, supports liver health, helps rid your body of any heavy metal toxins, and is necessary for the growth and repair of your intestinal lining. When starting off on L-glutamine, I suggest taking *half* the dosage recommended on the bottle, as your body needs to get used to this supplement. Take the half dose for two to four weeks and then increase to the full dose. My recommended brands are:

  Pure L-glutamine powder
  Leaky Gut Repair by Dr. Axe
  GI Renew by Chris Kresser

  Once you are feeling 85 to 90 percent better and most of your red-flag symptoms have subsided, you can cut back on or even remove this supplement from your diet. Continue with your regular consumption of bone broth for a great, naturally occurring source of L-glutamine. But you shouldn't be supplementing with this more than six to nine months.

- **Cod-liver oil:** I recommend supplementing with cod-liver oil because it is the richest source of omega-3 essential fatty acids (EFAs). These EFAs play an important role in helping our bodies produce and regulate hormones, manage inflammation, and maintain high-functioning brain, nervous, and immune systems. Omega-3 EFAs are commonly found in coldwater fish, flaxseeds, walnuts, legumes, nuts, and green leafy vegetables. Since the typical American diet contains more omega-6 EFAs (found in foods like grains, plant-based oils, eggs, and poultry) than omega-3s, and since a body in optimal health should have equal amounts, the key is to supplement with omega-3. In addition, cod-liver oil is a great source of vitamins A and D. Purchase this in capsule or oil form. The goal is to get in 1 teaspoon of cod-liver oil per day. If you experience loose bowel movements after taking it, cut the dosage back by half. The best high-quality, mercury-free brands I recommend are:

  Green Pasture's Blue Ice, high-vitamin cod-liver oil
  Carlson Lab's cod-liver oil

Rosita Extra Virgin Cod Liver Oil
NutraPro Virgin Cod Liver Oil

Ideally you will take 1 teaspoon daily (or the equivalent in capsules). However, if you have never taken this oil before, start with half the recommended dose and work your way up to the full dose. This is one of the supplements I recommend you take forever, because it's that good for you.

- **Liver:** Please note that liver is *different* than cod-liver oil; I want you taking liver *and* cod-liver oil. If you don't think eating 3 to 4 ounces per week of organic, grass-fed liver is going to happen, then I'd like you to take liver in capsule form. Liver is one of the best immunity-enhancing foods out there. The brands I recommend are:

  Dr. Ron's New Zealand grass-fed beef liver
  Vital Proteins Grass-fed Beef Liver

  Both these brands come in capsule form; take 1 to 2 capsules per day. And just as with cod-liver oil, I recommend taking liver for the rest of your life, or eating 3 to 4 ounces of grass-fed liver each week because it is that good for you).

This is the only vitamin/supplement regimen I want you to follow while you are doing the REAWAKEN phase of the *Body Belief* eating plan. Once you reach a point where your red-flag symptoms are gone, or at least 85 to 90 percent better, you can cut back on the digestive enzymes and the L-glutamine powder. I recommend keeping the probiotics, spirulina, liver, and cod-liver oil as a part of your daily regimen for life.

If you have a supplement regimen that is helping you manage a severe condition, discuss with your medical practitioner whether it's the right thing for your body to go off all your supplements. The goal here is for you to feel good, and if what you are currently taking has been helping you with a medical condition, then please discuss with your health-care practitioner before making any drastic changes. If you have specific questions related to your individual condition, or you are taking pharmaceutical medications, I recommend you discuss this protocol with your doctor or a healthcare practitioner.

To make this as easy as possible for you, I have created a sample seven-day REAWAKEN menu plan (Chapter 10) for you to follow so you can get the hang of the *Body Belief* eating plan. As well, head over to https://aimeeraupp.com/realplans for thousands of recipes that fit into the *Body Belief* eating plan. The RealPlans.com people have made healing from autoimmunity their full-time job and there are plenty of great recipes and meal ideas for you on their site.

Week Four

A Word on Reintroducing Food Groups

During the next several weeks of the REAWAKEN phase you will begin to slowly, week by week, reintroduce foods that were previously removed from your *Body Belief* eating plan. But keep in mind: this is a loose framework. You might do great following the REAWAKEN phase exactly as it is laid out, or you might need a different timetable that works for you. My recommendation to you is to reconnect to yourself and listen to how your body feels. Remember, reconnecting to yourself is one of the major points of this book.

If after the PURIFY phase and the first three weeks of the REAWAKEN phase you are still not feeling better or seeing improvements in your red-flag symptoms, then you should NOT begin reintroducing foods. Rather, you should stay with the foods you are eating until you see your symptoms begin to change for the better. If you begin reintroducing new foods too soon, you could set yourself and your autoimmunity back. So even though I have laid out the plan in a week-by-week fashion, I am leaving it up to you to stay attuned to how you're feeling and how your red-flag symptoms are improving, so you can best gauge when the right time is for your body to try new foods. Here's a rule of thumb: if after the PURIFY phase and the first three weeks of the REAWAKEN phase you are feeling about 80 to 85 percent better than before starting the *Body Belief* program, then you are ready to reintroduce new foods; otherwise give yourself a few more weeks before doing so.

After you make it through the first three weeks of the REAWAKEN phase, you will finally be able to try adding in some more food groups. But if you aren't yet seeing any major changes in how you feel or in your red-flag symptoms, then I want you to wait two more weeks before reintroducing any new foods. This goes for the remaining weeks of the REAWAKEN phase—you are going to be the best decision-maker as to whether to move forward with reintroducing new foods. Be sure to keep a detailed journal of how you are feeling, and how your red-flag symptoms are shifting and improving, so you can gauge when the best time is for your body to move forward with more food categories.

That said, if you are feeling great and have noticed that most of your red-flag symptoms have improved dramatically (yay you!), then you are ready to add nuts and seeds. But here is the key: they first need to be soaked in water and then dried before you can enjoy them. Soaking nuts and seeds before you eat them is imperative, as it helps break down phytates and phytic acids, enzymes that inhibit digestion and irritate your intestinal lining. Since your body is still in the healing process, the only way you can reintroduce nuts and seeds is to soak them and dry them first (p. 120); you can also find soaked (and often sprouted) nuts and seeds at your local health-food store—you can eat them as long as they are organic.

Do not add nuts or seeds to your diet any earlier than when I tell you, because they can cause a setback in your healing. If and when you add them, do so in moderation and specifically as I direct you: 1 tablespoon, two times a day for two consecutive days. This will enable you to see if there is any type of reaction to the food. If you eat the new food too far apart, meaning more than one day in between, you may not notice a reaction. Be sure to keep detailed notes on how you feel when you add them back in. If you get any digestive discomfort or a flare-up of any of your red-flag symptoms, or if you feel really tired, get a headache, or get an odd skin rash, you should wait another two weeks before trying nuts and seeds again or reintroducing any other new foods. If you don't feel any adverse reactions, then you can begin having these foods more regularly in your diet, but consume them in moderation: 3 to 4 tablespoons per week.

How to Soak Nuts and Seeds

What You Need

2 cups of raw, organic nuts or seeds (it is better to soak one kind at a time)

3 to 4 cups of warm filtered water (enough water to cover the nuts or seeds). *It's important that the water is warm.*

1 tablespoon of sea salt. (Salt is imperative to breaking down the phytic acid and phytates.)

What to Do

1. Place the warm water in a medium bowl or jar (half gallon or larger). Add the salt and let dissolve.

2. Add the nuts or seeds, making sure they are completely submerged in the water.

3. Leave uncovered on the counter or other warm place (not the refrigerator) for at least 7 hours, preferably overnight.

4. Rinse in a colander and spread on a baking sheet or dehydrator sheet. Bake in the oven at the lowest temperature (150°F is optimal, but 200°F will work too), or dehydrate until completely dry. This step is important, as any remaining moisture in the nuts or seeds can cause them to mold. Dehydrating time can often be up to 24 hours. A dehydrator simplifies the process but isn't necessary.

5. If you want to go one step further and make your own nut or seed milk, the best time to do it is right after soaking them, when the nuts and seeds are soft.

Week Five

By now you are really owning your new *Body Belief* eating plan and, if you would like, your body is ready to try coffee and alcohol again. When it comes to coffee, it is really important that you drink only organic coffee, and I want you to limit your intake to three to four cups per week maximum. With alcohol, I'd like you to limit yourself to two to three drinks per week maximum, always choosing a highly distilled spirit like vodka or tequila (and mixing it with something like fresh lemon or lime juice, or sparkling water). As with reintroducing the nuts and seeds, if you feel any adverse reaction to either the coffee or the alcohol, such as a headache or an upset stomach, or if you have trouble sleeping the night that you add it back in, coffee may not be for your body. But you can give it a try and see how you feel; be sure to take good notes.

Week Six

Your healing body is now ready to try another food group: fermented dairy products. If you've had dairy in the past and never had an allergic or anaphylactic reaction, then this week you can reintroduce grass-fed, full-fat fermented dairy in the form of yogurt, kefir, butter, or even a little cheese. (It is ideal if the cheese is raw; you can often find raw cheese at your local health-food store.) I repeat, these dairy products must be fermented, full fat, and grass-fed, as no other dairy will do. Just as with nuts and seeds, try two servings of fermented, full-fat, grass-fed dairy for two days in a row. You can mix them up, but don't do more than two servings in a day, and don't do more than two days in a row. Note how you feel. If you feel any digestive discomfort, get a headache or a skin rash, feel nauseous or tired, or experience a flare-up of any of your red-flag symptoms, stop the dairy and give your body a rest. Don't try dairy again for two weeks, and refrain from reintroducing any new foods. If you don't feel any negative reactions, then you can begin having these foods more regularly in your diet, but consume them in moderation: one to two servings per week.

Week Seven

This week we are going to hold off adding anything new to your *Body Belief* eating plan. Instead, we are going to focus on the following mantra: *My body is healing. I am whole.* I want you to practice this mantra daily, repeating it to yourself in front of a mirror.

Week Eight

Now you can, if you like, add back quinoa and rice. I would like you to hold off on any other grains for the moment, always keeping in mind that gluten should forever be out of your diet. The key with quinoa and rice, just as with nuts and seeds, is soaking them before you cook and eat them. The soaking makes them more digestible and decreases the drawbacks from the toxic lectins, phytic acid, and phytates.

How to soak quinoa or rice

What you need

2 cups quinoa or rice

2 cups warm filtered water

2 tablespoons raw apple cider vinegar

What to Do

1. In a glass or nonreactive bowl, mix the rice or quinoa with the warm filtered water and apple cider vinegar. Cover and let sit for 8 to 12 hours. (Note: you can soak the quinoa or rice longer than this, which is especially helpful if you have a history of five or more years of digestive issues. Just make sure you change the soaking water every 12 to 24 hours.)

2. When you are ready to cook the rice or quinoa, strain it in a fine sieve and rinse well, until the water runs clear. Make sure you thoroughly rinse quinoa, in particular; otherwise it can be bitter. Cook as usual.

Try having one serving of rice or quinoa two days in a row, and note how you feel. If you experience any negative side effects, discontinue the food and hold off adding any new foods for two weeks. If you don't feel any negative reactions, then you can begin having these foods more regularly in your diet, but eat them in moderation: one to two servings per week (of either quinoa *or* rice total; that is, one serving of quinoa and one serving of rice *or* two servings of one of them). Please note: It is not until you have been in the REAWAKEN phase for three months without any signs of your red-flag symptoms that I recommend trying quinoa pasta or brown-rice pastas.

Cookware and Storage: Avoiding Hidden Chemicals When You Cook

So you've made all of these amazing dietary and lifestyle changes, because you're ready for your own reawakened health. But what about all those sneaky chemicals hiding in your kitchen? I'm not talking about spray bottles under the sink. I'm talking about your pots, pans, and food-storage containers. Every time you heat a nonstick pan, you are leaking those chemicals into the air and your food. Every time you place your leftovers in a plastic (even BPA-free) container, you are putting yourself in danger. Here are my recommendations for safe and chemical-free cookware and food storage:

Cookware

Stainless steel: It's a classic and there's a reason. It's super clean. Stainless-steel pots and pans are great for cooking your meals. The only downside: they are not naturally nonstick, so they aren't great for a beginner cook. But with proper care, they can last a lifetime. The following brands make high-quality, nontoxic stainless-steel products:

Cuisinart   Calphalon   Cooks Standard   All-Clad

Cast Iron: A tried and true classic—these pots and pans have been used for cooking since the early 1700s and have been passed down from generation to generation. They are also naturally nonstick when properly seasoned, and have the benefit of being able to go from stovetop to oven to table very easily. The best brand (and the one I use at home) is:

Lodge

Enameled Cast Iron: These can also be kept for many generations, but have the downside of being a bit pricey. But they can often be found at yard sales or thrift stores with no loss of quality. These are my recommended brands:

Lodge   Le Creuset

Ceramic: These are super versatile, handle high heats like the cast-iron varieties, are naturally nonstick, and are easy to keep clean. The only downside? They *will* crack if dropped. These are not for the clumsy. The best brand is:

Xtrema

Stoneware: Looking to make the *perfect* pizza? This is your go-to. Stoneware just gets better with age. However, it is heavy and cumbersome. The best brand is:

Pampered Chef

Food Storage

Glassware is the best way to go for storage. Glass is so much easier to keep clean than plastic, and it doesn't get stained like plastic either. The possibilities are endless. A 12-pack of mason jars can be used as glasses or food storage (even for the freezer). There are many other glass food-storage options out there, but be wary of plastic lids. If you can't avoid plastic lids, be sure to let your food fully cool before putting them on, so condensation does not form on the lid and drip into your food. These are my recommended brands:

| Weck | MightyNest | Glasslock |
| Ball | Pyrex | VonShef |

Stainless steel is another great option, though it is not oven-safe, so you can't cook and store in the same containers. If you cannot avoid plastic lids, be sure to let food fully cool before putting them on, and avoid contact between the food and the lid. These are my recommended brands:

Klean Kanteen   Happy Tiffin   Lunchbots

Week Nine

At this stage, you have been following the *Body Belief* eating plan for a minimum of nine weeks! Congratulations! That is amazing! If you are moving along with reintroducing new foods, that tells me you are feeling good and your red-flag symptoms have abated. I am so excited for you and your thriving health. Now, if you love beans, it's time to try adding back some legumes (of course in moderation). As with grains and nuts and seeds, you need to soak the legumes before consuming them. Here's what you do:

- For kidney-shaped beans, add enough water to cover the beans and a pinch of baking soda. Cover and allow them to sit in a warm kitchen for 12 to 24 hours, changing the water and baking soda once or twice.

- For non-kidney-shaped beans such as northern beans or black beans, place beans into a pot and add enough water to cover the beans. For every 1 cup of beans, add 1 tablespoon of apple cider vinegar.

- If you are soaking legumes, it is best to rinse them several times during the soaking time to prevent them from starting to ferment (this is a food group you do not want to eat fermented, as it can be toxic). Always rinse legumes before cooking.

- After soaking is done, rinse the beans, replace the water, and cook for 4 to 8 hours on low heat or until beans are tender.

When reintroducing, try one serving of soaked and cooked beans two days in a row, and note any reactions you may have. If you have any major reactions, such as a headache, a skin rash, or digestive discomfort, discontinue the beans. But if you feel good after eating them and none of your red-flag symptoms flare up, then you can add legumes to your diet in moderation, one to two 2-ounce servings per week.

Week Ten

Your healing body is now able to try some nightshade vegetables. Since there are quite a few of these vegetables, I want you to pick your three favorite ones and try reintroducing them one at a time. Do just what you did with the other foods you reintroduced, trying the food two days in a row, noting any reactions, and then waiting four days and repeating with another nightshade vegetable. Most people at this stage will do well with eggplant and sweet peppers, while some will also be OK with chili peppers and white potatoes. Most of you still won't feel great eating raw tomatoes, but cooked ones may be fine.

Week Eleven

If you miss egg whites, here is the week to try whole eggs. If you have eaten eggs in the past without any major allergic or anaphylactic reaction, and you've been doing fine with egg yolks in your *Body Belief* diet thus far, you can give whole eggs a try. You can reintroduce egg whites by having two whole eggs per day for two days in a row. Doing it this way will allow you to see if your body is having a reaction to egg whites. (Note: if you've been feeling good eating just the yolks, you can keep up with the one to two yolks per day recommendation.) Take the time to really reconnect with yourself and note how your body feels after adding back in the egg whites. If you have any reactions such as a skin rash, headache, digestive discomfort, or a flare-up of any of your red-flag symptoms, you need to discontinue the egg whites for now, but you can try again in two weeks. In the meantime, hold off adding any other new foods.

Week Twelve

You must be feeling great! Your body is now ready for some of my favorite indulgent foods: gluten-free flours! This means you can start making some yummy gluten-free muffins and pancakes. The flours I want you to stick with are blanched almond flour, coconut flour, arrowroot powder, and tapioca starch. With these four ingredients you can begin to make all sorts of yummy treats. You can now also try, a few times each week, adding 1 to 2 teaspoons of raw cocoa (in powder or nib form) and raw honey (be sure it's raw, as it's best for your immune system), and seeing how you feel. Take it easy and introduce this group of foods slowly. By no means are you to overdo it with gluten-free pastry goods; limit yourself to one serving per week.

OK, we have just covered a *lot* of information. You now have a three-month *Body Belief* eating plan that will help you reconnect with yourself, renew your beliefs, and reawaken your health. One thing I want to emphasize is that you stick to the first 30 days of this diet as best you can. When you do this plan exactly as I have laid out, you will give your body and its cells the best opportunity to thrive and heal. Truly committing to the first 30 days of the *Body Belief* eating plan will help reduce inflammation in your body, regulate your immune system, heal your gut lining, and repair any damaged parts of your body that were victims of autoimmune attacks. That said, some of you may need 60, 90, or even 180 days before your body really begins to heal. That's why the most important piece to this entire *Body Belief* program is to reconnect to yourself, so you can hear the cues from your body and know what is right for your healing path.

You will see major improvement in your health following this protocol, but no matter what, I want you to do what feels right for you and your body—mentally, emotionally, physically, and nutritionally. Ideally you will always limit your intake of grains; soak the nuts, seeds, and beans you eat, and consume them in moderation; consume pseudograins only once in a while, if at all, if they're well tolerated by your body (or if the side effects are worth it). If you never liked beans to begin with and don't miss them at all on this diet, then you don't need to add them back in. If you don't feel well eating as much fat as I recommend, then gradually introduce more fat into your diet while listening to your body's needs. If drinking bone broth for three solid days doesn't resonate with you, then modify the plan to something that does resonate with you (while sticking to eating only the *Body Belief* foods). And if after following this protocol you want to indulge in gluten or conventional dairy or soy—that's your decision. Just note what I said about these foods and how they affect inflammation and autoimmunity in your body. The risks these foods pose are very real.

Bottom line: reconnect to you so you know how to best serve your body and its health, because every *body* is different, and every autoimmune disease is different. What I have laid out for you is a framework, or a guideline. Follow it as best you can while being aware of your body and its needs. And if you need more help and guidance on this path, reach out to me for private coaching or find a good functional-medicine practitioner that you can work with. My recommendations are not a cure; they are a pathway to your healing. Your body and its condition may need more one-on-one work, but the *Body Belief* plan is a great jumping-off point. It will pave the way for your health transformation.

OK, now it's time to dig into even more ways you can REAWAKEN your health.

Chapter Nine

C

Reawaken Your
Health a Little More

Now that you have the *Body Belief* eating plan down, you are ready to tackle another very important piece of your health transformation: your personal beauty and home-care products. Food is only one part of the reawaken phase; the other part is how you interact with your physical environment. From what you put on your skin to the quality of the air you breathe to how much or how little you exercise to how much time you spend in nature to the quality of your sleep—all of these environmental things matter because they impact your health and your immune system.

From a TOM perspective, your interaction with your external environment affects the quality and the abundance of your qi. Qi is one of the vital substances for life, and it is derived from the foods we eat and the air we breathe.

It is widely acknowledged that the air you breathe should be fresh, clean, and non-toxic (and that you should be getting out into nature on a regular basis). But because the skin is your largest organ, it literally breathes in everything it comes into contact with. So the next step in your health reawakening process is to remove the toxic chemicals from your environment, especially from your skin.

Toxins in Your Personal-Care Products

The average woman "wears" nearly five hundred chemicals each day by way of such things as makeup, body lotion, face cream, hand lotion, deodorant, toothpaste, nail polish, shampoo, perfume, hair product, sunscreen, household cleaning supplies, laundry detergent, and dish soap.[1] Many of these chemicals have been linked to everything from hormonal imbalances to cancer to autoimmune conditions. Yes, every personal-care product that your skin comes into contact with can exacerbate your autoimmune condition. Chemicals in your environment are involved in your autoimmunity.[2] Over the last four decades, close to one hundred thousand chemicals have been introduced into our environment, many of them finding their way into our personal care. On top of that, the Food and Drug Administration (FDA) does not investigate or test for the safety of personal-care products, leaving you subject to harm by an overabundance of toxic chemicals.

So, what does this mean for you?

Not only are nonorganic, pesticide-ridden foods compromising your health, but so, very likely, are the personal-care, beauty, and body products you are using. In order to truly transform and reawaken your health, you must completely avoid the following 15 ingredients:

1. Fragrance (a.k.a. artificial fragrance, synthetic fragrance, parfum, perfume): This is used to make things smell good, but it is a scientifically proven hormonal disruptor.[3] Look for products that are labeled "fragrance-free," and use essential oils to make things smell nice.

2. Sulfates (Sodium Lauryl, Sodium Laureth Sulfate (SLS) and Sodium Lauryl Ether Sulfate [SLES]): These are foaming agents, and they make things lather up. They are usually found in toothpaste, shampoo, body washes, and soaps. These noxious substances are skin irritants, hormone disruptors, and carcinogenic. Also,

be wary of labels that say "Sodium Lauryl Sulfate (derived from coconut oil)": they may be phrased to look like they're natural and non-toxic, but the way they make coconut oil into SLS is through a highly chemical toxin-producing process. Buy only products that are sulfate-free.

3. Butylated hydroxyanisole (BHA) and butylated hydroxytoluene (BHT): these two chemicals are common preservatives in moisturizers and makeup (and a lot of packaged food products). They are carcinogenic, cause thyroid problems, and have been shown to cause reproductive disorders.

4. Parabens (methyl, propyl, butyl, and ethyl): We all know to avoid parabens, right? These guys are the worst. These endocrine-disrupting chemicals (EDCs) are used to preserve products for longer shelf life. They are also very disruptive to our hormones and immune system. Many believe parabens play a significant role in male *and* female infertility. They also have harmful implications in developing children, and have been tied to the higher incidence of breast cancer and autoimmune conditions.[4] Avoid parabens at all costs, period.

5. Polyethylene glycol (PEG, PEG-20): This stuff is actually used in oven-cleaner products as a powerful degreaser and is used in industrial antifreeze. PEG has been linked to kidney damage, leukemia, breast cancer, uterine cancer, and brain cancer.[5] People handling it are warned by the manufacturer to avoid skin contact and wear respirators and rubber gloves, yet this is a major ingredient in most moisturizers, skin creams, baby wipes, and sunscreens. You will also find it in many skin cleansers, shaving cream, lip balm, and even contact solution and laxatives! Why? It's cheap and gives the "glide" factor in body

lotions, but it is in fact robbing moisture from lower layers of skin. Lanolin and collagen also clog pores and cause skin to age faster than if nothing was used. Go PEG-free.

6. Phthalates (a.k.a. benzene, DEP, DBP, DEHP and any word that has "phth" in it): These noxious EDCs are a family of industrial plasticizers already banned in the EU from being used in plastic toys, but are still in hairs prays, perfumes, and nail varnishes. They can be absorbed through the skin, inhaled as fumes, and ingested from contaminated food or breastfeeding. Go phthalate-free.

7. Formaldehyde (a.k.a. DMDM hydantoin, diazolidinyl urea, imidazolidinyl urea, methenamine, and quaternium-15.): When combined with water, this toxic gas is used as a disinfectant, fixative, germicide, and preservative in deodorants, liquid soaps, nail varnish, and shampoos. Also known as formalin, formal, and methyl aldehyde, it is a suspected human carcinogen and has caused lung cancer in rats.[6] It can damage DNA; irritate the eyes, upper respiratory tract, and mucous membrane; and may cause asthma and headaches. It is banned in Japan and Sweden.[7]

8. Toluene: a common solvent found in nail enamels, hair gels, hair spray, and perfumes. It is a neurotoxin and can damage the liver, disrupt the endocrine and immune systems, and cause asthma.

9. Talc: A known carcinogenic that has been linked to an increased risk of ovarian cancer and general urinary-tract disorders. Don't dust it on your baby's, or anyone else's, bottom!

10. Oxybenzone (a.k.a. benzophenone, ethoxycinnamate, and PABA): This sunscreen chemical will not only disrupt your hormones but also damage DNA and lead to certain cancers.

11. Diethanolamine (a.k.a. Tri and Mono, DEA, TEA, and MEA): An EDC that is used in creamy and foaming products, this toxin is absorbed through skin and has been shown to be carcinogenic.

12. Aluminum: This is most commonly found in deodorants and has been linked to diseases such as Alzheimer's and breast cancer.

13. Triclosan (a.k.a. 5-chloro-2-[2,4-dichlorophenoxy] phenol): This antimicrobial, antibiotic agent is found in hand sanitizers, deodorants, toothpastes, vaginal washes, and mouthwashes. It has been found to negatively affect the thyroid, the immune system, fertility, and fetal development, and can lead to an increased risk of miscarriage.

14. Petrolatum (a.k.a. mineral oil, petroleum): A known carcinogen that is used to make products slick and moisture-rich, it's found in everything from hair spray to shampoo to mouthwash. Avoid it.

15. Bisphenol A (BPA): This chemical is produced in large quantities primarily for use in the production of polycarbonate plastics and epoxy resins. Typically this is found in food and drink packaging, such as water and infant bottles, impact-resistant safety equipment, and medical devices; but it can be found in packaging for all types of products, including home and beauty products. Epoxy resins are used as lacquers to coat metal products such as food cans, bottle tops, and water-supply pipes. Some dental sealants and composites may also contribute to BPA exposure. Go for products packaged in glass *or* plastic, and in tin packaging that says BPA-free.

I'm sure this list is a lot to digest. So here are the top things you need to do to rid your personal care routine of these harmful chemicals:

- Take an hour and read the labels of *all* products that come in contact with your skin, and toss the products that contain any of these chemicals.

- Take a look at the list of *Body Belief*–approved products (p. 203) and try some of them out.

- If tossing all of your personal-care products is cost-prohibitive, start slowly and replace one per week or one every other week. Bottom line: you need to stop using toxic products, as they are not serving your health; nor will they allow the radical healing your body is capable of.

- Download these two apps: Think Dirty and Healthy Living. These two apps allow you to scan the barcode of any personal-care product for a ranking of its toxicity level. My general recommendation is to stay below a two for any product you let touch your skin.

- Consider keeping it simple. Use coconut or olive oil for your skin lotion. Use ghee or coconut oil as your facial moisturizer (I use a mixture of both!). Use coconut oil as your facial cleanser (it works so well!). Use baking soda for your toothpaste and arrowroot powder as your deodorant. Use brown sugar or sea salt for exfoliating your skin. Use liquid castile soap as the only soap in your home (I even make my son's baby wipes with Dr. Bronner's castile soap and olive oil). For household cleaning, apple cider vinegar and baking soda are the only two products you'll ever need. Or do what I did and start making your own products using different carrier oils and essential oils. Consult the list of *Body Belief*–approved products you can use (p. 203), as well as my DIY recipes for personal-care and household-cleaning products (p. 211).

There are definitely a lot of products out there that we can use and feel good about it, but just because something says "all natural" or "organic" doesn't mean it's free of toxic chemicals. The way I see it, if you can't eat it, you shouldn't be putting it on your skin. Another thing to beware of: many companies change their ingredients regularly, so please always read labels.

Next, I want to discuss with you three very important pieces to recovering and reversing the damage done to your body from the many years of being exposed to environmental toxins.

Reversing the Damage of Environmental Toxins

Throughout this book I have given you the tools to shift your emotional, physical, and nutritional state, so that the immune attack against you and your body will recede and you can transform your health for the better. Now I want to talk to you about three crucial lifestyle factors that influence and impact your health:

1. Sleep

2. Movement

3. Nature

The *Body Belief* framework that you now have will, when followed closely, help you change your health for the better. But your body's optimal functioning is also dependent on how much (or how little) you sleep, how much (or how little) you move, and how much (or how little) you interact with nature. If you don't sleep enough, your body will never have all the resources it needs to heal or to regulate its immune system; nor will it be able to efficiently utilize the resources you provide it with. If you don't move enough, nothing will flow in your body and your qi will get stuck, making healing a challenge. And if you aren't connected to the ebbs and flows of nature and your external environment, it will be tough for your body to find the balance it needs to thrive.

From one of the oldest extant texts of TOM, *The Yellow Emperor's Classic of Internal Medicine,* written around 300 B.C., comes some wisdom that will help you truly embrace all aspects of your healing path:

> Qui Bo replied, "In the past, people practiced the Tao, the Way of Life. They understood the principle of balance, of yin and yang, as represented by the transformation of the energies of the universe. They formulated exercises to promote energy flow to harmonize themselves with the universe. . . . They ate a balanced diet at regular times, arose and retired at regular hours, avoided overstressing their bodies and minds, and refrained from overindulgence of all kinds. They maintained well-being of body and mind; thus, it is not surprising that they lived over one hundred years.
>
> "These days, people have changed their way of life. They drink wine as though it were water, indulge excessively in destructive activities, drain their *jing*—the body's essence that is stored in the kidneys—and deplete their qi. They do not know the secret of conserving their energy and vitality. Seeking emotional excitement and momentary pleasures, people disregard the natural rhythm and order of the universe. They fail to regulate their lifestyle and diet, and sleep improperly. So it is not surprising that they look old at fifty and die soon after."

Take in those words and understand that the information in this book is a guide for finding your way again, so that you can learn to live in accordance with the laws of the universe, and to love, respect, and honor the vessel that is your body. All that said, here are three more things you need to be doing to reawaken your health:

1. Sleep seven to eight hours every single night. If you have trouble sleeping, get yourself to journal and meditate more, use blackout shades or an eye mask,

and remove all electronics from your bedroom. Bedrooms should be for sleeping and sex, so that means no television or electronics in the bedroom.

2. Move daily. Moderate exercise seems to be the best for those dealing with and healing from autoimmunity (that's you!). Try a stretching routine, walking, yoga, Pilates, cycling, or hiking for 30 to 40 minutes at minimum three to four times per week. Have a dog? Walk it! Have friends who cycle? Join them. Too cold to leave your home? Have a dance party in your living room! Are there woods behind your home? Go exploring! Keep in mind we are aiming for daily, *moderate* movement. Intense cardio may be too much for your body right now. Reconnect to yourself and see how your level of activity feels to you. If you aren't doing enough, move more. If you are exercising a lot and feel exhausted, cut back. But do something every day.

3. Reconnect to nature. Sunlight and fresh air are crucial to the healing process. They stimulate immune function, regulate your hormones, and cultivate healthy, abundant qi. Make it your business, no matter the weather, to get outside every single day and breathe in fresh air. If you live near a park or a forest, or have a backyard filled with trees, go there and take a walk. And weather permitting, walk around barefoot in the grass and get in some unprotected sunlight. Yes, *unprotected* sunlight, ideally—for 10 minutes twice per day.

And because I want your health to transform in miraculous ways, I have a few more tools and tips you can incorporate into your life to maximize your healing journey. My recommendation is to try the tools that resonate with you the most. If anything I recommend or that someone else recommends feels good to you, and you believe it could help improve your health, try it. If it doesn't feel good to you, hold off.

As you're learning these tools, listen to your body and feel your reaction. If you feel excited, curious, or a sense of ease, then the tool could be good for you. Alternatively, if you feel tense or uneasy or find yourself rolling your eyes, then it isn't the right time for that tool. Reconnect to you so you can listen to and hear what your body needs. Honor how you feel and what resonates with *you*.

Yoga and Mudras for Autoimmunity

To bring you the best of what yoga can offer for the management of autoimmune disease, I teamed up with my dear friend and peer, Karon Shovers Goldsmith. *(NOTE: If yoga is not for you due to injuries or other concerns, sitting in a comfortable position and breathing works too. You can do just that as your pose, and it counts.)* Karon has been practicing yoga for over 20 years and has used her practice as a means to heal her body after suffering a stroke at the age of 23. Her passion is helping women to find balance in their hurried lives, inviting them to connect to their very own life force (you can learn more about Karon at KaronShovers.com).

Here is the protocol Karon and I designed for you. As we see it, combining gentle low-impact yoga, breathing, and meditation creates a perfect formula for helping people with autoimmune diseases and inflammation disorders. Yoga can address some of the emotional and physical challenges brought on by autoimmune disorders. It can also improve range of motion, reduce fatigue, and promote a state of relaxation that can reduce the stressors that compromise the immune system. (Also, if you want to see this protocol and more autoimmune yoga in action, check out the video Karon and I made for you on AimeeRaupp.com/bodybelief.)

Four Core Yoga Poses

1) *Tadasana* (Mountain Pose)

Physical benefits: Increases balance, endurance, and concentration. This pose requires effort each time it is done. The yogi strives to quiet the mind and focus on the breath while holding the pose, breathing quietly for 30 seconds to one minute at a time.

Emotional and spiritual benefits: Tadasana will help you feel calm, centered, and steady. When you feel grounded, you can reconnect to your body with a more positive attitude.

Instructions: Stand with your feet shoulder-distance apart. Balance the weight evenly on all four corners of your feet (big toe mound, inner heel, little toe mound, outer heel). Balance evenly on right and left feet. Look straight ahead, finding a point (*drshti*) at eye level to focus on. Soften your shoulders and let your arms rest at your sides, palms facing each other. Feel the ground supporting you and breathe.

This pose is the foundation for all standing yoga poses. Once you have mastered Tadasana and feel strong and stable in the pose, you can move on to the hundreds of other standing variations.

2) *Virabhadrasana* II (Warrior Pose II)

Physical benefits: Strengthens and stretches legs, torso, and arms. Can relieve leg cramps, revitalize abdominal organs, and increase respiration and circulation. This pose can assist your body with managing stress and functioning effectively.

Emotional and spiritual benefits: Helps you feel grounded, powerful, and clear about your true purpose.

Instructions: Start in Tadasana (see above), widen your feet about four feet apart. Raise your arms parallel to the floor, palms facing down. Extend arms from midline, stretching through elbows, wrists, and fingertips, keeping your shoulder blades going back. Turn your right foot out 45 degrees, and keep your left foot parallel to the back of the mat. Bend your right knee, making sure the knee is over the ankle and moving toward the second toe. Make sure the weight in your feet is even on the front foot and back foot. Repeat on left side. Breathe. Start at 10 seconds on each side and work yourself up to 30 seconds on each side.

3) Supine Twist

Physical benefits: This pose is good for digestive health, which is connected to your immune system response and inflammation. This pose will release tension in the lower back and shoulders. The internal organs will compress and squeeze, bringing fresh blood and oxygen into the organs.

Emotional and spiritual benefits: Twists are cleansing, and literally wring out the internal organs, which helps your body release old energy, leaving space for new delight and a higher purpose.

Instructions: Lying down on your back, bend your knees with your feet on the floor, and allow your knees to fall to your right side. Keeping your knees together, allow your left shoulder to release to the floor. Support your left shoulder with a folded blanket or towel if it does not reach the floor easily. To intensify this pose, you can place your right hand on your left thigh, grounding the thigh to the floor. Breathe. Start at 10 seconds on each side and work yourself up to 30 seconds on each side.

4) *Viparita Karani* (Legs-up-the-wall pose)

Physical benefits: This pose inverts the typical actions that happen in our bodies when we sit and stand. Lymph and other fluids that accumulate in swollen ankles, tired knees, and congested pelvic organs are allowed to flow into the lower belly. This refreshes the legs, abdominal organs, and reproductive area. It also increases blood flow to the upper body and head, which creates a sense of balance and renewal. Roger Cole, Ph.D., did research on inversions and found they alter hormone levels, which can decrease brain arousal, blood pressure, and fluid retention.[8]

Emotional and spiritual benefits: Helps us remember that positive results can come from doing less, not more. This restorative pose helps you practice the polar opposite of activity, which is receptivity, so you can be open to receiving your highest self. Heightens your sense of well-being and ease.

Instructions: Place the long side of a bolster (or folded yoga blanket with a six- to eight-inch fold) parallel to the wall. Sit on one end of the bolster and simultaneously swing your legs up the wall, placing your head and shoulders on the floor. If this is difficult, try it without the bolster. Your legs and torso will make a right angle. This should be relaxing. If there is too much stress on the legs or hamstrings, you can microbend your knees. *Caution: this pose is not recommended for people who should avoid inversions due to retinal problems, menstruation, hiatal hernias, or eye-pressure disorders.*

Two Key Mudras for Inflammation and Autoimmunity

Mudras are hand gestures. Most mudras can be done by anyone, regardless of physical mobility.

Anjali Mudra (gesture of offering)

Instructions: Join together the right and left palms in front of the heart. You can touch your thumbs to your heart center. As you hold this mudra, repeat the following mantra: I step into my power as I love, forgive, and honor my body.

Physical benefits: As a centering gesture, it can help you feel focused and calm. It can also increase flexibility in hands, wrists, fingers, and arms.

Emotional and spiritual benefits: The act of doing this mudra provides a connection between the right and left hemispheres of the brain, and connects the practitioner with their highest self. It is an honoring of the self and the divine within us. This mudra can assist in meditation.

Prithvi Mudra (gesture of the earth)

Instructions: Place both palms face up and rest on thighs in a seated position. Connect the thumb and ring fingers of both hands. Gently extend the other fingers. Relax the hand. As you hold this mudra, repeat the following mantra: I am connected, I am rooted, and I am healing.

Physical benefits: This mudra builds and invigorates organ tissues and strengthens the bones. It increases the earth element in the body but decreases the fire element, which is at the core of inflammation and pain.

Emotional and spiritual benefits: It can produce a sense of stability, confidence, and strength, which helps us to feel compassion for ourselves and others.

Acupuncture and Chinese Herbs

We have discussed TOM quite a bit, but I haven't mentioned much about acupuncture or Chinese herbs yet. That is not because I don't practice acupuncture and see clinical results with it, or don't prescribe Chinese herbs and believe they are extremely powerful substances, because I do. I have seen firsthand the clinical effects of both these modalities, and how they can help improve your health, your body's healing, and the management of autoimmunity. In fact, I highly recommend you work with an acupuncturist and/or Chinese herbalist on your path to reawakened health.

Both acupuncture and Chinese herbs have been used for centuries to improve blood flow and circulation in the body, regulating a person's immune system and decreasing inflammation. Acupuncture regulates immune function, enhances anti-cancer and anti-stress immune function, and regulates anti-inflammatory pathways in the body. Acupuncture and moxibustion (another tool we use regularly in TOM, by which mugwort, an herb, is burned to improve circulation and blood flow) have profound benefits for immunity.[9] According to TOM, there are over a thousand acupuncture points on the body; these acupuncture points are areas of the body that influence the flow of qi and energy when manipulated by acupuncture needles or acupressure). One acupuncture point in particular, Stomach 36, has been shown to protect the intestinal mucosal immune barrier; specifically, it "attenuates the systemic inflammatory response through protection of intestinal barrier integrity . . ." What that means is that this acupuncture point can help with treating leaky gut or intestinal permeability.[10]

Many studies have looked into the far-reaching effects of acupuncture on health and healing, and researchers using functional MRI (magnetic resonance imaging) have found that the insertion of these tiny needles affects the body on the hypothalamus-pituitary-adrenal axis level, indicating that acupuncture works via the nervous system to regulate the stress response, immune function, and hormone and inflammatory pathways.[11] Put simply, acupuncture is one of the best modalities one can use when dealing with an autoimmune condition.

Be sure you find a practitioner who has extensively studied acupuncture and Chinese herbology, and is certified by the National Certification Commission for Acupuncture and Oriental Medicine (NCCAOM). You also have the option of working with me online, or if you're in the New York City area, you can come into one of my clinics and work with me or one of my associates. In the meantime, I want to share with you two helpful acupressure points that you can start using right now to help regulate your immune system.

1. Stomach 36 (*Zu San Li*): This acupuncture point is commonly used for any gastrointestinal discomfort. It was also taught to me as being one of the great points for boosting vitality and immune function. Additionally, there is research showing its effectiveness in helping with immunity and the healing of intestinal permeability.

    Location: It is found four finger-widths down from the bottom of your knee cap, along the outer boundary of your shin bone or the lateral part of your lower leg. Place your hand at the bottom of your kneecap. When your pointer finger is touching the bottom of your kneecap, your pinky finger will fall right on Stomach 36. If you are on the correct spot, a muscle should flex as you move your foot up and down. Once you find the point, use medium pressure (as if you're pressing a thumbtack into a soft corkboard) to massage in a clockwise motion (as if your body is the clock) for one to two minutes. Repeat on the other leg. You can do this twice per day to activate this acupuncture point and boost your immune system.

2. Lung 7 (*Lie Que*): The lung channel in TOM is the one most closely associated with the immune system. Activating Lung 7 can help fight off a cold or flu, but it can also help keep the immune system strong, so you can avoid getting sick. I find this acupressure point particularly effective if the person has grief or sadness associated with their immune condition.

Location: Keep your hand with the nail of your thumb pointing up toward the ceiling. Move your thumb up and back (away from the palm of your hand), which will reveal a depression at the bottom of the thumb, which is called the "anatomic snuffbox" (between two tendons). Move your finger from the anatomic snuffbox up the side of your lower arm, about 1.5 inches, until you feel a bone sticking out. Lung 7 is located on that bone, in between the two tendons you feel there. Apply acupressure by pressing this point with your thumb or index finger in a clockwise motion (as if your body is the clock) for one to two minutes. Repeat on the other arm.

Applying acupressure on Stomach 36 and Lung 7 on a daily basis will help regulate your immune function. For more effectiveness, find a local NCCAOM-certified acupuncturist to work with.

When it comes to specific Chinese herbal treatments for your specific symptoms, an NCCAOM board–certified Chinese herbalist can make an individualized formula just for you. Chinese herbs are prescribed according to specific herbal properties, such as acupuncture meridian entered, functions, clinical use, major combinations and dosage. Don't worry if it sounds complicated; board-certified Chinese herbalists keep up with the current pharmacological research on Chinese herbs, including their potential drug interactions; antimicrobial, antiviral, and antifungal effects; and effects on blood pressure, smooth muscle, hormones, the central nervous system, and gynecology.

Only go to a qualified and NCCAOM board–certified acupuncturist and herbalist for treatment. Be smart and check out the credentials of any and all medical professionals from whom you seek advice. Unfortunately there are practitioners who are not as qualified to treat you as they should be. And *do not* self-treat with Chinese herbs. Just because they are natural, they shouldn't be self-prescribed. Please seek herbal advice from someone who is trained in using them and understands any and all potential interactions they may have in your body.

Emotional Freedom Technique (EFT)

EFT, or "tapping," is a form of acupressure where you tap or activate certain acupuncture points while you think about, voice, and work through an ailment or—better yet—a belief you are ready to renew. As an acupuncturist, I find the method of EFT fascinating—it's basically a psychological acupressure session where you can help your body let go of any emotions you are holding on to. Not only does the act of tapping acupuncture points while voicing aloud a stressful belief help you work through a negative belief and release it, but it has also been scientifically shown to reduce the stress hormone cortisol and alleviate anxiety levels.[12]

Qi Gong

Qi Gong is a series of slow meditative movements combined with deep breathing and focused concentration; it has been an integral part of TOM for thousands of years. You may have seen it in the movies or maybe in your local park, as many Chinese-American communities will practice Qi Gong daily. It is often recommended by TOM practitioners as an exercise to improve health and vitality. Through using breath with coordinated movements, this technique cultivates qi in your body, supports the functioning of your immune system, improves circulation and blood flow through your entire body, and is an amazing stress reliever. Practicing Qi Gong can help you breathe new life into your body and support your healing process by simply inhaling and exhaling.

The following two Qi Gong exercises are said to improve qi flow in your body, promote healing, and boost the three substances vital for fertility: qi, blood, and essence. It is said that it is best to practice Qi Gong from 7 to 9 A.M., or 7 to 9 P.M. outside in nature—but for now you should practice it wherever and whenever you can. The more you practice these exercises, the more you will be in touch with the natural rhythm of your body, your qi, and how your qi flows through your body. These exercises are yet another way for you to reconnect to you.

1. *Open Your Heart*

   Instructions: Stand with feet shoulder-width apart and swing your arms at your sides up to the height of your mouth. Swing them in unison. Do this for at least three minutes. While you are swinging your arms, concentrate on energy flowing through your chest and your heart, opening your heart to letting go of any anxiety and tension. While practicing, repeat this mantra: *I am letting go of tension and opening up to receive my wellness.*

2. *Invigorate Your Essence*

   Instructions: Take the palms of both your hands, place them over your kidneys (located on either side of your lower back, right above your hip bones) and begin to rub them back and forth. As you rub, focus on the connection between your palms and your kidneys. The palms are associated with your heart, and by rubbing your palms over your kidneys you are creating a circuit between the heart and kidneys. Your heart is connected to the emotion of joy, and your kidneys to the emotion of courage. Do this for at least three minutes, focusing on sending strong and joyful energy through your body. While practicing, repeat this mantra: *I am joy. I am strength.*

Functional Medicine

Similarly to how TOM is practiced, functional medicine works to identify and solve the root problem of a health concern. Functional-medicine practitioners are health-care practitioners who have completed additional training in patient-centered treatments. That means that rather than treating isolated symptoms, as many Western medical specialists do, functional-medicine practitioners look at the whole patient to understand how genetics, lifestyle factors, nutrition, and environmental factors can influence health.

As an acupuncturist and herbalist with a strong background in Western medicine, I can interpret my clients' lab results and guide them to the proper medical tests to have done so we can figure out what exactly is going on in their body and how to rectify it. But not all acupuncturists practice like this, and not all health-care practitioners practice like this.

For you, having a health-care professional who can understand all sides—Western medical lab results, alternative approaches, nutrition, and mind-body—can propel your health forward faster. That's how I work, and that's how many practitioners trained in functional medicine and nutrition work. For you, these types of doctors are the best kind to work with, because an integrative approach is what your body needs. These practitioners are health detectives and consider *all* factors of your life and your medical history in order to get to the root cause of your condition. They will look at your lab test results for functional ranges—these ranges are different from the lab range. For example, if a patient gets their thyroid tested, and the results of the TSH (thyroid-stimulating hormone) are 3.5 mlU/L, their Western doctor will likely tell them that their thyroid levels are normal, since the "normal" range for TSH is between 0.45-4.50 mlU/L. This is quite a wide range, but if you fall somewhere within that range, purely Western doctors will likely tell you all is well. I myself or a functional-medicine practitioner would disagree, because the functional range (by this I mean, the range at which your body and its organ systems function optimally) for optimal TSH levels is between 1 and 2 mlU/L. Furthermore, most Western doctors wouldn't do a complete thyroid panel to see how *all* the thyroid hormones are functioning, but a practitioner who is looking to treat the root of the disease would, *because all the thyroid hormones really matter.*

I know you want to find the best support for yourself on your path to health and vitality. My recommendation: schedule an online consult with me or find a like-minded practitioner to work with, such as a functional-medicine doctor, nutritionist, or health-care practitioner. It is important to your healing process to work with a health-care professional who can treat you holistically, since an integrative approach is what your body needs. In my opinion, the best referrals come from trusted sources like friends or family who have had success working with the practitioner. But you could also find someone who practices functional medicine or functional nutrition by going to the Institute for Functional Medicine website (FunctionalMedicine.org) or to paleophysiciansnetwork.com. In addition, here are some tips on recognizing the practitioners who will best support you on your new *Body Belief* path:

- They recommend a diet and lifestyle very similar to what is laid out in this book. A well-trained practitioner will understand the *Body Belief* approach, and agree that you should be following this plan (or a very similar one) for a minimum of one to three months.

- They specialize in autoimmune disease. You need to work with someone who understands autoimmunity.

- They don't promise a cure or remission. Unfortunately, there is no cure for autoimmunity, but you can heal your body. If someone promises you a cure, I'm not sure you should trust them. Your health can heal, and it will, but there will be ebbs and flows. What you want is a better quality of life, and for your red-flag symptoms to radically improve. This book alone can help you get there, but finding more support may be beneficial as well.

- They see themselves as part of a team. You want to work with someone who really listens to every detail and who understands what is going on with you and your body. You want someone who sees your health rejuvenation as a team effort. No health protocol is a one-size-fits-all type of thing.

- They are not "over-supplementers." You do not need to be on a million supplements. In fact, you should be on only a few, and they should all be food-based and made with super-clean ingredients.

- They are paying attention to your symptoms and adjusting treatment accordingly. Your health routine is going to be different from everyone else's, since everyone heals differently. You want to work with someone who understands that, and is in touch with how your health is shifting, so they can adjust protocols accordingly.

- Avoid working with practitioners who do any of the following:

    - Tell you that diet doesn't matter
    - Recommend you buy a dozen supplements before leaving their office

- Don't discuss the benefits of bone broth and healing a leaky gut
- Want to put you on a juice cleanse
- Don't listen to you
- Make you feel powerless

You can get the following lab tests done if you want to find out more about your autoimmunity; your regular doctor may order these tests for you, but you will often need to work with a functional-medicine doctor to get these tests completed. *(Note: not everyone needs all of these tests, but I want to point them out as they can give you even more information.)*

- Comprehensive Blood Test—You likely already get this test done annually. But just as I described with regard to the TSH scenario, the kind of practitioner you work with should be looking out for functional ranges, *not* just normal ranges.

- Comprehensive Stool Test—Work with a practitioner who can recommend and interpret this type of test, which will screen for parasites and pathogens as well as beneficial bacteria and the health of your intestinal lining. From my research and clinical experience, the best lab to test the health of your gut is Doctor's Data.

- Urine Organic Acids Test—This test will tell your practitioner a lot about what is going on with your body's metabolism and cellular function. Recommended labs for these tests are Genova and Great Plains.

- SIBO Breath Test—SIBO stands for "small intestine bacterial overgrowth," which is common in autoimmune conditions and digestive disorders, and can be a serious condition if left untreated. It is helpful for practitioners to do this test to learn more specifics, so they know how to treat you if you have. The recommended lab for this test is Genova.

- Hormone Testing—Your hormones are directly linked to your autoimmunity, and getting them tested is super important. However, standard blood work just won't do enough. You need to get hormone testing through your urine. (Saliva is another good way, but there is a new urine test called the DUTCH test that is even more accurate than saliva.) Be sure you are getting a *complete* thyroid panel, including TSH, Free T3 and Free T4, reverse T3, and thyroid antibodies. *All* of these tests should be done on your thyroid, and if your doctor doesn't think they are all necessary, find a new doctor, because your thyroid should be looked at and your doctor should support your requests.

- 23andMe—You can now order a saliva test online from 23andMe.com, and the test will tell you a lot about your genetic predispositions to certain diseases and disorders. Of course, you know that it's epigenetics and how you live your life that determine whether these genes get turned on. But by finding out your genetic predispositions, you can support your body and its health even more. Order the "ancestry" test and then use a site like MetabolicHealing.com to have the data interpreted for you. You can use the 23andMe site to interpret your results, but I have found that MetabolicHealing.com offers you a more in-depth interpretation at a cheaper price. Of course, you can also choose to leave the decision and interpretation up to your health-care practitioner. But keep in mind: this test should not be used for diagnostic purposes; rather, it is to be used as a means of understanding your genetics risks and predispositions. It is *not for medical diagnoses.*

You can order most of these tests yourself online or through a site like DirectLabs.com, but your health-care practitioner should be able to order them and interpret them for you. Again, not all of these tests are necessary, but they can give you more information about what is going on in your body. I recommend that you check with your health insurer to see if you can get these tests covered when ordered by your health-care practitioner.

The tests you do *not* need to do (and which are a waste of your money) are IgG blood tests for food sensitivities, IgE food-allergy blood tests, food-intolerance testing, heavy-metal testing, and leaky-gut testing (you are already treating your leaky gut with the *Body Belief* protocol, so you don't need an expensive test). If your doctor pushes you to get these tests done, question why.

I hope this information will help you get even farther along your path to reawakening your health and truly heal. I have shared these tools and recommendations with you so that you can have even more ways to maximize your healing process. But that doesn't mean you have to do all the things I've listed. Some may resonate with you, and some may not. The ones that don't resonate with you now may resonate with you later. Healing and reawakening your innate vitality takes time, and you will need different things at different times. No matter what, continue to stay reconnected to you, and to the place where you will make the best decisions for your body and its health.

In the next chapter, I am going to outline a 7-day *Body Belief* plan, covering everything from what and when to eat, to "food gratitudes," to recipes, to meditations and more! You have laid the groundwork. Now let's make the *Body Belief* plan a part of your normal routine!

Chapter Ten

Body Belief in Action: 7-Day Plan

This 7-day *Body Belief* in Action plan will be your general weekly guide as you continue on the lifelong REAWAKEN phase of the *Body Belief* plan. This 7-day plan should be started *after* you complete the 11-day PURIFY phase (p. 104). My intention is to give you a framework for how your new *Body Belief* way of life will look. Of course you can adjust where needed for your lifestyle and recipe preferences, but know that the 10 basics of the *Body Belief* in Action plan should be implemented so you can see the results you are longing for.

Always remember:

You are worthy of thriving, you are worthy of having fewer red-flag symptoms, and you are worthy of more energy and clearer thoughts. You are ready to feel better and heal your body. I believe in you and your body and your cells and your ability to feel better, and I hope you do too.

Here are the basics of the *Body Belief in Action* plan:

1. Get seven to eight hours of uninterrupted sleep each night.

2. Eat within the first 30 minutes of waking up and eat every two to three hours after that.

3. Reconnect to yourself daily—through meditation, journaling, breathing, or whatever helps you to reconnect—so you can hear the conversation you are having with yourself.

4. Practice the A.R.T. of Shifting Your Beliefs (p. 59) as often as you can. (Remember, A.R.T. stands for Acknowledge, Renew, and Transform.)

5. Get moderate exercise, 30 minutes, four to five days each week.

6. Be easy on yourself. Cheer yourself on more than you don't; be understanding and compassionate toward *you*.

7. Drink good-quality water throughout your day.

8. Take your supplements every day (p. 114).

9. Be conscious of the food you eat and how it nourishes your body.

10. Pick one day a week to prepare your meals ahead of time. It will make this whole process so much easier.

Bonus: Take a few moments each day and send love to the 37 trillion cells in your body—you can do this through meditation, journaling, or simply stating to yourself, "To all the cells in my body, I love you and I thank you for supporting my health transformation."

The 7-day *Body Belief in Action* plan

This plan is based on a *7 A.M.* wake-up and an *11 P.M.* bedtime, but adjust it your schedule as needed.

Day One

7 A.M.: Wake up and say to yourself, "Today is a new day, and I deserve to feel good."

7–7:05 A.M.: While still in bed, take 10 long and slow deep breaths, tuning in to your body. Notice any thoughts that pop into your head; and after you take your 10 deep breaths, note the thoughts or beliefs that came up for you in your journal so you can work through those thoughts. P.S. You are reconnecting to yourself and it feels good.

7:20 A.M.: Before you begin preparing your breakfast, make yourself some hot tea (organic green or black) with juice from half a lemon, *or* have a mug of hot water with juice from half a lemon or a tablespoon of apple cider vinegar.

7:30 A.M.: Breakfast: two scrambled egg yolks with spinach and fresh parsley, a piece of bacon, and ¼ of an avocado. Before you eat, repeat your food gratitude of the day: *Thank you for nourishing the 37 trillion cells in my body.*

7:45 A.M.: Take a look in the mirror and say something kind to yourself, such as "You are doing great; I am proud of you."

7:50–8 A.M.: Prepare your lunch and snack for the day and put it in a stainless steel or glass to-go cup (see p. 123 for the best food-storage containers).

10 A.M.: Snack: ½ cup of organic blueberries mixed with 1 tablespoon of Vital Proteins Collagen Peptides, 2 ounces of full-fat coconut milk, and 2 ounces of water. Blend it and make a mini-smoothie! *Tip: You can double this recipe and have half for your morning snack and half for your late afternoon snack.*

11:30 A.M.: Get outside for a quick five- to ten-minute walk to soak in some sunshine, even if it's super cold or super warm out. Just go!

12:30 P.M.: Lunch: The Ultimate Prebiotic Salad topped with sautéed wild halibut (p. 198). Before you eat, repeat your food gratitude of the day: *Thank you for nourishing the 37 trillion cells in my body.*

12:45 P.M.: Practice some pranayama breathing (p. 45), and be sure to hydrate with good-quality water.

3 P.M.: Snack: the other half of your morning smoothie.

4 P.M.: Reconnect: What are you saying to yourself right now? Do you notice any running conversations you're having with yourself? Write them down.

6 P.M.: Dinner: One 4-ounce baked chicken breast with fresh herbs, sautéed kale with garlic, and a sweet potato with one teaspoon of ghee. Share mealtime with a friend or loved one, and find time to laugh. Before you eat, repeat your food gratitude of the day: *Thank you for nourishing the 37 trillion cells in my body.*

7 P.M.: State this renewed belief to yourself: *I am ready to feel better.*

9:30 P.M.: 4 ounces of Golden Turmeric Sipping Broth (p. 177); just a little nibble to keep your blood sugar even while you sleep.

10 P.M.: "Lights out," meaning all electronic devices off, and start getting ready for bed. Spend time in your bedroom writing out one of your "I Am" statements 10 times, such as: *I am healing.*

11 P.M.: Time for sleep.

Bring Nature Inside:

Grow a garden and fill your house with plants. Science shows that indoor plants boost moods, reduce anxiety and depression, and improve air quality.

Day Two

7 A.M.: Wake up and notice how cozy your bed is or how rested your body feels. Look around your room. Could you make some changes—a new fluffier pillow, organic sheets, inspiring photos, pictures of something or someone that makes you smile, or just decluttering so your bedroom feels more like a sleeping sanctuary?

7–7:03 A.M.: Red-flag check-in: how are your symptoms feeling so far today? Rate your top three red flags on a scale of 1 to 10 (1 meaning, "they are barely bothering me," and 10 meaning, "I feel terrible today").

7:20 A.M.: Make yourself some hot tea (organic green or black) with juice from half a lemon, *or* have a mug of hot water with juice from half a lemon or a tablespoon of apple cider vinegar, *or* make yourself a cup of the Liver Support Juice (p. 196. Note: don't have this juice more than four times per week).

7:30 A.M.: Breakfast: Yolkocado (p. 188). Before you eat, repeat your food gratitude of the day: *Food is my greatest medicine and I love the food I choose to nourish my body with.*

7:40 A.M.: Take five minutes to be mindful: sit and breathe, journal, or take a walk in nature.

7:55 A.M.: State aloud a renewed belief, such as, *I do feel better when I take better care of myself.*

10 A.M. Snack: 4 ounces of coconut-milk kefir and an apple *or* grapefruit.

11 A.M.: Reconnect: What are you saying to yourself? Be honest with yourself and then be kind to yourself.

12:30 P.M.: Lunch: 2 organic grass-fed sausages (pork or turkey) sautéed in 1 tablespoon of a healthy fat, 1 cup of roasted veggies (such as brussels sprouts and beets). Before you eat, repeat your food gratitude of the day: *Food is my greatest medicine and I love the food I choose to nourish my body with.*

1 P.M.: Reconnect: How is your body feeling right now after lunch?

3:30 P.M.: Snack: 2 cups of cut-up melon with 1 tablespoon of gelatin sprinkled on it, *or* ½ cup of sauerkraut and a handful of plantain chips. Eat slowly and enjoy the nourishment.

5:30 P.M.: Get out for a moderately vigorous walk. If you're at work, sneak out for a "coffee break" and get in 15 to 20 minutes of walking.

6:30 P.M.: Dinner: 3 ounces of pan-seared beef tenderloin with sautéed spinach, brussels sprouts, Jerusalem artichokes, and garlic. Flavor with juice from half a lemon and a dash of sea salt. Before you eat, repeat your food gratitude of the day: *Food is my greatest medicine and I love the food I choose to nourish my body with.*

8 P.M.: Snack: 4 ounces of bone broth. Sip slowly and feel its healing properties.

9:30 P.M.: Spend some quality time doing something you love: reading a book, cooking your food for tomorrow, knitting, watching your favorite TV show or movie, taking an Epsom-salt bath, making love with your partner or to yourself (yes, I said that!). Just do something that feels good and nurturing to you.

10 P.M.: Turn off all electronics. Take a few minutes to work on your Good Journal entry (p. 67); contemplate the good in your life.

11 P.M.: Bedtime.

Day Three

7 A.M.: Wake up and check in: how are you feeling? Find one thing that feels good to you right here, right now.

7–7:10 A.M.: Spend a few minutes and reconnect to you through breathing or journaling. Then spend some time checking in with your red-flag symptoms and how they're improving (you can use the feeling-tracker tool on p. 64).

7:20 A.M.: Make yourself some hot tea (organic green or black) with juice from half a lemon, *or* have a mug of hot water with juice from half a lemon or a tablespoon of apple cider vinegar.

7:30 A.M.: Breakfast: coconut-milk smoothie: 2 to 3 ounces of full-fat unsweetened coconut milk (you can also use almond milk if you prefer), ½ avocado, ½ cup of raspberries or strawberries, 1 tablespoon of Vital Proteins Collagen Peptides, 1 tablespoon of MACA powder, and 2 to 3 ounces of water (depending on how you like your shakes). *Tip: Double the recipe and drink half for breakfast and the other half as your snacks for today.* P.S. Don't forget your food gratitude for the day: *I lovingly chew and digest my food, allowing its nutrition to heal me.*

7:55 A.M.: Take a moment to state a renewed belief: *There's no harm in making the Body Belief dietary changes that Aimee recommends.*

10 A.M.: Snack: some of your leftover smoothie from breakfast, *or* an apple with coconut butter.

11 A.M.: Reconnect: what are you saying to yourself? I hope it's something nice. If it's not, add a compliment to your self-talk.

12 P.M.: Sneak a look in the mirror. While looking into your own eyes, say to yourself, "I am well."

1 P.M.: Lunch: watercress salad with grilled chicken or salmon, with cooked and diced beets, broccoli, olive oil, and vinegar. Flavor with some fresh ground pepper and Himalayan sea salt. Be sure to say your food gratitude for the day: *I lovingly chew and digest my food, allowing its nutrition to heal me.*

2 P.M.: Get outside for a few minutes. Or at the very least, spend some time seeing and feeling and being present in the environment around you. How do you feel?

3:30 P.M.: Snack: the rest of the morning smoothie *or* an Epic Bison Bacon Cranberry Bar (p. 201).

4 P.M.: Note your red-flag symptoms. How are they doing: worse, better, or the same?

6:30 P.M.: Dinner: Pan-sautéed filet of sole with shallots and leeks, and sautéed kale and asparagus with rosemary (all cooked in a healthy fat). Add the juice from half a lemon. Be sure to say your food gratitude for the day: *I lovingly chew and digest my food, allowing its nutrition to heal me.*

7:30 P.M.: Spend 20 minutes doing the autoimmune yoga sequence (p. 138) because the 37 trillion cells in your body deserve it.

8 P.M.: Do nothing. Give your mind and body a real rest. No electronics, no TV, no noise. Nothing.

8:30 P.M.: Snack: Sip on 4 ounces of bone broth or have two Chocolate Coconut Power Balls (p. 193).

10 P.M.: All electronics off. Take a few minutes to write down the five things in your Good Journal (p. 67).

11 P.M.: Bedtime. As you're lying there in the quiet, repeat to yourself a kind thought: I am doing the best I can do with what I have available to me.

Day Four

7 A.M.: Wake up and check in with yourself. How are you feeling? How is your body feeling? Did you have any dreams last night? Can you find a few things that you feel good about right now?

7–7:03 A.M.: Write down a few things that feel good to you right now.

7:20 A.M.: Make yourself some hot tea (organic green or black) with juice from half a lemon, *or* have a mug of hot water with juice from half a lemon or a tablespoon of apple cider vinegar, *or* make yourself a cup of the Liver Support Juice (p. 196; Note: don't have this juice more than four times per week).

7:30 A.M.: Breakfast: Bone Broth Egg Drop Soup (p. 176). Take time to eat slowly and repeat your food gratitude for the day: *My food soothes my immune system.*

7:55 A.M.: Sneak a glance in the mirror and say something nice to yourself, such as, "I am proud of you."

10 A.M.: Snack: ½ cup of Fermented Veggie Medley (p. 173) in 4 ounces of Golden Turmeric Sipping Broth (p. 177) *Tip: prepare 8 ounces and drink half now and half later.*

11 A.M.: Get some fresh air or spend some time staring out at nature, even if it's only the plant in your office.

12:30 P.M.: Lunch: grilled or sautéed fish of your choice, with sautéed spinach over a fermented red-cabbage slaw. Garnish with cracked pepper and pink Himalayan sea salt. Take time to eat slowly and repeat your food gratitude for the day: *My food soothes my immune system.*

1 P.M.: Connect with someone (a loved one, a best friend, a valued coworker) who makes you feel good and/or who has been kind to you recently. Send them a thank-you note or return the compliment.

3:30 P.M.: Snack: the rest of the Golden Turmeric Sipping Broth (p. 177).

4:30 P.M.: Take a few minutes to do some pranayama breathing (p. 45) or a quick yoga pose (pp. 139–141).

5:30 P.M.: Smile at a stranger; or if that's not working for you, smile at yourself in the mirror. Remember: kindness heals.

6:30 P.M.: Dinner: three turkey meatballs or any other meat you choose (about 4 ounces of meat in total) over zoodles or spaghetti squash in No-Mato sauce with a side of sautéed veggies (p.

189). Take time to eat slowly and repeat your food gratitude for the day: *My food soothes my immune system.*

8:30 P.M.: Do nothing. Relax. Send love to your body's cells.

9 P.M.: Snack: a handful of blueberries with some coconut kefir.

10 P.M.: All electronics off. Spend time doing something you love, such as stretching, breathing, reading, crosswords, playing a musical instrument, or drawing or cuddling with your partner.

11 P.M.: Bedtime. As you're falling asleep, repeat an "I Am" statement, such as: *I am vital.*

Kindness Heals

Science shows that being kind to others—in the form of a gift or a compliment or a charitable contribution—increases health benefits in those with chronic illnesses. (http://link.springer.com /article/10.1007%2Fs10902-011-9267-5#page-1)

Day Five

7 A.M.: You are awake! It's a good day! Find one thing to be grateful for.

7–7:05 A.M.: Reconnect: How are you feeling? Take a few moments to check in on your red-flag symptoms. As always, it's a good day to feel good.

7:20 A.M.: Make yourself some hot tea (organic green or black) with juice from half a lemon, *or* have a mug of hot water with juice from half a lemon or a tablespoon of apple cider vinegar.

7:30 A.M.: Breakfast: Golden Turmeric Sipping Broth (p. 177). Don't forget your food gratitude of the day: *I appreciate my ability to feed myself healing foods that have been made with love.*

7:50 A.M.: Spend 20 minutes doing the autoimmune yoga sequence, or do deep breathing and visualizing yourself healthy and strong, because the 37 trillion cells in your body deserve it.

10 A.M.: Snack: ½ cup of Organic Gemini Tiger "Nuts" (p. 201) and a banana.

11 A.M.: Sneak a look in the mirror, and while looking into your eyes say something kind like "You are healing."

12:30 P.M.: Lunch: sautéed shrimp with garlic and leeks topped with 1 ounce of fish roe, served over cauliflower rice. Don't forget your food gratitude of the day: *I appreciate my ability to feed myself healing foods that have been made with love.*

1:30 P.M.: Get some nature time. Leave your smartphone behind and take in a dose of fresh air, and think about a renewed belief. Here's an example: *My body is programmed to thrive, and I am supporting it.*

3:30 P.M.: Snack: ½ cup of sauerkraut and a handful of parsnip chips.

4 P.M.: Take five minutes to be mindful: sit and breathe, journal, or take a walk in nature.

6:30 P.M.: Dinner: a bunless burger topped with avocado, pickles, and homemade horseradish sauce, served with half a baked yam topped with cultured ghee and sea salt. Don't forget your food gratitude of the day: *I appreciate my ability to feed myself healing foods that have been made with love.*

8:30 P.M.: Be kind to yourself and relax in whatever way works for you (maybe even a cocktail of top-shelf vodka with fresh-squeezed lime juice and seltzer water).

9:30 P.M.: Snack: A handful of plantain chips with half a cup of Fermented Peach Chutney (p. 172).

10 P.M.: Slip into some cozy pj's and get ready for bed. If you have a partner, say something nice to him or her.

11 P.M.: Bedtime.

Day Six

7 A.M.: Wake up and reconnect. How are you feeling? Find one good thing about your body; even the tiniest thing counts.

7–7:05 A.M.: Spend five minutes meditating. Your mantra could be something like, "My cells love me and I love them back."

7:20 A.M.: Breakfast: Yolkocado (p. 188) and a glass of the Liver Support Juice (p. 196; Note: don't have this juice more than four times per week). Eat slowly and repeat your food gratitude of the day: *All is well with my cells.*

7:45 A.M.: If you have time, spend 20 minutes doing the auto-immune yoga sequence (p. 138) or get outside for a brisk 20-minute walk. You can even do something more high-intensity like cycling or swimming, if that's available to you.

10 A.M.: Snack: Epic Bison Bacon Cranberry Bar (p. 201).

11 A.M.: Make sure to have a good belly laugh; free YouTube videos are great for this.

12:30 P.M.: Lunch: coconut-milk yogurt with fresh berries. Eat slowly and repeat your food gratitude of the day: *All is well with my cells.*

2 P.M.: Take a moment to journal about what's going on in that mind of yours. Remember: your body hears everything your mind says.

3 P.M.: Snack: 4 ounces of bone broth (pp. 180–187) with coconut milk.

4:30 P.M.: Practice a renewed belief, such as, "I'm getting better every day."

6:30 P.M.: Dinner: pan-sautéed pork chops with your favorite veggies. *Eat slowly and repeat your food gratitude of the day: All is well with my cells.*

8:30 P.M.: Do something fun tonight: go out with your partner or a good friend. Or just take some time to dance in your house to your favorite song. Enjoy this beautiful life you are living. If you feel unwell, I promise listening to a fun song or an '80s dance hit will lift you, if only for a few minutes. And those few minutes count.

9:30 P.M.: Snack: two or three Chocolate Coconut Power Balls (p. 193).

10 P.M.: All electronics off. Spend time doing something you love like reading or cuddling with your partner.

11 P.M.: Bedtime. Night, night.

Gratitude Heals

Numerous studies have shown that practicing gratitude decreases depression, improves health and well-being, benefits relationships, and decreases pain and suffering. So practice gratitude, daily!

Day Seven

7 A.M.: Wake up and say to yourself, "Today is a new day and I deserve to feel good."

7–7:05 A.M.: Red-flag check-in: how are your symptoms feeling so far today? Rate your top three red flags on a scale of 1–10.

7:10 A.M.: Make yourself some hot tea (organic green or black) with juice from half a lemon, *or* have a mug of hot water with juice from half a lemon or a tablespoon of apple cider vinegar.

7:20 A.M.: Breakfast: Scrambled egg yolks with avocado and bacon. Eat slowly and repeat your food gratitude of the day: *My food heals me.*

7:35 A.M.: Take 20 minutes to do some yoga, trampoline rebounding, or brisk walking.

10 A.M.: Snack: 4 ounces of Golden Turmeric Sipping Broth (p. 177) *Tip: prepare 8 ounces and drink half now and half later.*

11 A.M.: Tell someone in your life why you are grateful for them. It can be anyone—your mail carrier, your mother-in-law, your doctors, yourself!

12:30 P.M.: Lunch: tuna salad with plantain chips. Eat slowly and repeat your food gratitude of the day: *My food heals me.*

1 P.M.: Connect with nature. Get outside for 10 minutes, no matter the weather.

3 P.M.: Snack: kombucha and a pear with coconut butter.

4:30 P.M.: Practice a renewed belief: I know in my heart I am meant to feel better than I do now.

6:30 P.M.: Dinner: Your favorite protein (fish, poultry, or meat) sautéed with your favorite veggies. Cooked, of course, in a healthy fat. Eat slowly and repeat your food gratitude of the day: *My food heals me.*

7:30 P.M.: Snack: A handful of plantain chips with some guacamole.

8 P.M.: Start a batch of homemade bone broth (pp. 180–187).

8:30 P.M.: Say something kind to yourself and to whomever else is with you. Then watch a show or read a book that makes you laugh.

10 P.M.: Get out your Good Journal (p. 67) and note some things that are good in your life.

11 P.M.: Bedtime. Sleep tight!

There you go! Seven days of the *Body Belief* plan all laid out for you. As I said, all of the recipes I mentioned in your new *Body Belief Action Plan* are included in the back of this book. In addition to recipes, I've also shared some on-the-go snack ideas that you can buy pre-made to make your life even easier. Now you are ready to dive into your new *Body Belief* way of living and completely reawaken your health.

Chapter Eleven

Believing in
the New You

I am so honored to be at this place with you—the place where you are ready to own your new *Body Belief* way of life. I know that I have given you a lot of information. I also know you're doing your best to follow my advice and honor your body. It is my hope that you're reconnecting to yourself on a daily basis, or as often as you can; and that from that place, you're beginning the process of renewing your beliefs and hearing what it is you are saying to yourself in private. But most importantly, it is my desire that through all of this, *you* are being kind to *you*.

Be easy on yourself, because the *Body Belief* plan is a lifestyle overhaul and not a quick fix. Take all of this in at your own pace; follow the *Body Belief* plan in a way that feels good to you, and know that even the smallest attempts at nurturing and honoring your body will support your healing path. You are doing the best you can from where you are, and you're doing great. So take a deep breath, reconnect to you, and know that you are ready for more wellness and less suffering.

Your body hears everything your brain says. Your thoughts rewire your brain and affect your physiology. And now you have the tools to hear and shift the conversation you are having with yourself, so that you can truly allow your health to thrive. You are now armed with new strategies to acknowledge, renew, and transform your body beliefs because you understand how your beliefs dictate your behavior and therefore dictate your life choices. Your eyes are now open to the fact that the mind-body component is the cornerstone of your healing transformation. You are ready and willing to reconnect to yourself and renew your beliefs, as often as you can, because you want to feel better. You know you deserve to feel better. You are stepping into the well-being you are worthy of, and you are cheering yourself and your cells on more than you're not.

If there is only one thing you take from the *Body Belief* lifestyle, I hope it is the sheer importance of you being kind to you, and finding compassion for yourself and where you are. There's more and you're ready for it—you're excited to have a new way of eating because it feels good to know that food can nourish and support the cells in your body. It feels good to know that you are eliminating toxins from your emotional, nutritional, and physical life because you are aware of how harmful they are to your health, and there's no turning back. You are propelling your health forward and are eager for more energy, more comfort, and more wellness. The *Body Belief* lifestyle is in you, and you are radically shifting your health and loving your body more.

Even if you're not wholly there yet, or even halfway, that's OK, because you are closer than you were when you started. Even if you follow these teachings only most of the time, you are going to see results. We are all human, and everyone has their own pace for change. The goal is for you to become rooted in self-love and respect, because once you're in that place the lifestyle and diet changes will flow. When you make choices and decisions from a place of self-love, it will be simple to allow your health to thrive, because you will choose to do only what feels good on every level.

If all you do right now is work on the reconnecting piece of the *Body Belief* plan, getting to know yourself and your body again, then I feel I have done my job. I want you to happily and gracefully inhabit your body and mind again. I want to see you living from a place of forgiveness, kindness, and compassion for yourself. As you do that, the shifts will unfold, and deciphering what feels right for your body will be automatic. From a place of self-love, it will be easy to avoid toxins in your life—from toxic relationships to toxic foods to toxic exposures—because you will have great respect and admiration for the mighty being that you are, and for the awesomeness of the cells in your body.

I have been in the business of healing for a long time, and here's what I know for certain: when you are reconnected, you heal. When you are honest with yourself, kind to yourself, forgiving of yourself, lighthearted with yourself, and grateful for where you are *now*, radical changes happen. We can all commit to a two-week diet, new supplement regimen, or meditation practice for a certain period of time—but without being rooted in self-love and reconnecting to ourselves, the commitment will fade. That's why the first pillar of the *Body Belief* plan is: reconnect to you. From that place of being reconnected, you will renew your beliefs *just like that*. And when the renewal takes hold and the beliefs shift to kinder ones, you reawaken. And through it all, you will begin to notice your red-flag symptoms shifting, your energy improving, and a feeling of being more alive and believing in your body.

Of course you will have setbacks; that's normal and to be expected. But the difference is that, gradually, the setbacks won't last as long, you'll recover more quickly, and you'll get back to the place of hope faster.

So take a deep breath. Know that you can heal your body. Know that you can feel better. And know that you sure as heck deserve to. One day at a time, reconnect with yourself and tune into the cues from your body while practicing self-love and being easy on yourself. By embracing the *Body Belief* plan, you will radically transform your health!

I will forever believe in you and your ability to thrive!

All my love and gratitude to you.

Xo,
Aimee

Recipes

SIMPLE SAUERKRAUT

Yield: 3 to 4 servings

Ingredients

4 or 5 heads of red or green cabbage, shredded
¼ cup sea salt

Directions

1. Place the shredded cabbage little by little in a fermentation jar (a large, wide-mouth mason jar works great), pounding it vigorously and sprinkling some with the sea salt as you go.

2. Make sure that the mixture fills up the jar to no more than 1 inch below the top (because of the expansion; add more if needed), and that the extracted water covers the vegetables entirely. If it doesn't, create your own brine of 2 tablespoons sea salt and 4 cups water, and add it to the cabbage.

3. Press the cabbage and keep it under the brine. Cover with a clean towel or cheesecloth to keep out fruit flies. (It is important not to cover with a lid, because you need the airflow but don't want bugs.)

4. Place the fermentation jar in a warm spot in your kitchen and allow the sauerkraut to ferment for 7 to 10 days. Check on it from time to time to be sure that the brine covers the vegetables, and remove any mold that may form on the surface. Taste the sauerkraut during the fermentation process, and move it to the refrigerator when you're satisfied with the taste.

VINEGAR TONIC

Yield: 1 serving

Ingredients

2 tablespoons raw organic apple cider vinegar
½ teaspoon maple syrup
7 ounces seltzer

Directions

1. Grab an 8-ounce glass and put in vinegar and maple syrup. Fill the glass the rest of the way with seltzer.

FERMENTED PEACH CHUTNEY

Yield: 3 to 4 servings

Ingredients

16 peaches, cored and chopped coarsely
2 cups raisins
2 ½ tablespoons sea salt (plus 2 more tablespoons if extra brine is added)
Juice of 5 lemons
4 onions, finely chopped
4 tablespoons fresh ginger, grated

Directions

1. Combine the peaches with the raisins, sea salt, lemon juice, onions, and ginger.

2. Place the mixture little by little in a fermentation jar (a wide-mouth mason jar works great!), pounding it vigorously to release the juices.

3. Make sure the mixture fills up the jar to no more than 1 inch below the top (because of the expansion) and that the extracted water covers the mixture. If it doesn't, create a brine of 2 tablespoons sea salt and 4 cups water and add it to the mixture.

4. Press the mixture and keep it under the brine. Cover with a clean towel or cheesecloth to keep out fruit flies. (Do not cover with a lid because the airflow is necessary for fermentation.)

5. Place the fermentation jar in a warm spot in your kitchen and allow the chutney to ferment for 2 to 4 days. Check on it from time to time to be sure that the brine covers the vegetables, and remove any mold that may form on the surface. Taste the chutney during the fermentation process, and move it to the refrigerator when you're satisfied with the taste.

FERMENTED VEGGIE MEDLEY

Yield: 3 to 4 servings

Ingredients

4 organic apples, cored and diced
4 cups organic cauliflower florets
4 organic carrots, peeled and diced
8 green onions, sliced thinly
3 tablespoons fresh ginger, grated
½ cup sea salt

Directions

1. Combine the apples, cauliflower, carrots, onions, and ginger.

2. Place the mixture little by little in your fermentation jar (a wide-mouth mason jar works great!), sprinkling some of the sea salt as you go.

3. Make sure the mixture fills the jar up to no more than 1 inch below the top (because of the expansion). If it doesn't, create a

brine of 2 tablespoons sea salt to 4 cups water and add it to the mixture. Cover with a clean towel to keep out fruit flies.

4. Place the fermentation jar in a warm spot in your kitchen, and allow the mixture to ferment for 3 to 5 days. Check on it from time to time to be sure that the brine covers the mixture, and remove any mold that may form on the surface. Taste the veggie medley during the fermentation process, and move it to the refrigerator when you're satisfied with the taste.

COCONUT-MILK YOGURT

Yield: 2 to 3 servings

Ingredients

1 BPA-free can of full-fat coconut milk, 13.5 ounces (Native Forest organic is great)

1 tablespoon Inner-Eco fermented coconut-water probiotic kefir, or 1 capsule of any probiotic to use as your starter

½ teaspoon of organic ground cinnamon

Directions

1. For thicker yogurt, refrigerate the can of coconut milk (don't shake it up) for at least 3 hours so that the cream rises to the top. Then use just the cream, not the water, at the bottom of the can. If you prefer a thinner yogurt, use the entire can of coconut milk—water and all. The amount of yogurt you get from this recipe is equal to the amount of coconut milk you use. So if you use an entire 13.5-ounce can, you'll get the whole 13.5 ounces, or about 1 ¾ cups.

2. Place the coconut milk, or just the cream if you choose, into a sterilized glass jar with either the tablespoon of kefir or the contents of the probiotic capsule. If you're working with the probiotic capsule, open it up and dump in the powder. Then mix with a plastic or metal spoon.

3. Put the sealed jar of yogurt in the oven with the light on. DO NOT TURN THE OVEN ON. Just close the oven door and turn on the oven light. A closed oven with the light on will generate a stable temperature of about 105° to 110°F, perfect conditions for the coconut milk to incubate. The longer it sits, the more yogurt-y it becomes, so I leave mine in for 24 hours. Normally, you'd let dairy milk sit for 7 hours after heating it up on the stove to get it to that 110°F, but I'm using a shortened preparation process. It's not necessary to heat up either dairy milk or coconut milk before letting it incubate. The yogurt may still be watery; if so, put it in the refrigerator for a few hours to help it solidify. Before eating, sprinkle with cinnamon.

COCONUT-MILK KEFIR

Yield: 2 to 3 servings

Ingredients

Activated milk kefir grains (preferably from CulturesForHealth.com)
13.5 ounces of full-fat organic coconut milk (I like the brands Native Forest and Let's Do Organic)

Directions

1. Place the milk kefir grains in coconut milk. Stir with a non-metal spoon.

2. Cover with a coffee filter or cloth, secured by a rubber band.

3. Let it sit at room temperature, 68° to 85°F.

4. After 12 hours, begin checking the coconut-milk kefir every few hours, up to a maximum of 24 hours. Remove the milk kefir grains once the coconut kefir reaches the desired consistency.

Note: Sometimes kefir grains will require an adjustment period, so the first batch of coconut-milk kefir may not culture as desired. Use the coconut milk from this batch for cooking, and place the milk kefir grains in fresh coconut milk. An adjustment period isn't uncommon whenever kefir grains are switched from one type of milk to another (cow to goat, pasteurized to raw, dairy to coconut, etc.).

Milk kefir grains can be cultured in coconut milk regularly but should be revitalized in dairy milk for 24 hours once every few batches.

Dehydrated milk kefir grains should be rehydrated and fully activated in dairy milk before being used to culture coconut milk.

BONE BROTH EGG DROP SOUP

Yield: 1 to 2 servings

Ingredients

2 cups bone broth

1 egg yolk

¼ teaspoon ginger, minced

1 tablespoon spinach, coarsely chopped

1 tablespoon scallions, finely chopped

¼ teaspoon salt

Directions

1. Heat the broth until rapidly boiling.

2. While the broth boils in a small bowl, whisk one whole egg if you're eating both the yolk and the white. If you're eating just the yolk, then whisk only the yolk.

3. Drizzle the egg slowly into the boiling broth, while mixing it in with a fork. The egg should cook immediately.

4. Add ginger, spinach, scallions, and salt, and simmer another 1 to 3 minutes until the scallions are soft. Serve warm!

Note: Some mornings when I'm in a rush, I just add a whisked egg yolk, a handful of spinach, and a few dashes of sea salt to boiling bone broth—and it's delicious.

GOLDEN TURMERIC SIPPING BROTH

Yield: 3 to 4 servings

Ingredients

4 cups chicken broth
1 cup full-fat coconut milk (I like the brands Native Forest and Let's Do Organic)
1 teaspoon ground turmeric
1 teaspoon ground ginger
2 to 4 cloves of garlic, smashed and peeled
Pepper, freshly ground
Sea salt

Directions

1. Combine all the ingredients in a medium saucepan and bring to a low simmer.

2. Simmer on low or medium-low heat for about 10 minutes. Remove from the heat, salt to taste, and drink up!

YUMMY BUTTERNUT SQUASH SOUP

Yield: 5 to 6 servings

Ingredients

32 ounces organic butternut squash, cut into 1-inch cubes
4 tablespoons cultured ghee

Sea salt
Freshly ground black pepper
1 large yellow onion, chopped
3 cloves garlic, minced
5 cups bone broth
Fresh cilantro, chopped, for garnish
½ avocado, diced, for garnish

Directions

1. Preheat the oven to 400 degrees. On a foil-lined pan, toss the butternut squash in 2 tablespoons of ghee and a pinch of salt and pepper. Roast in the oven for 15 to 20 minutes (depending on the size of the cubes) until the squash is tender. Use a fork to test how tender it is.

2. In a large pot, add the remaining 2 tablespoons of ghee and onion, and sauté over medium-high heat for about 10 minutes until the onion has softened. Add the garlic and sauté for an additional minute.

3. Add the roasted butternut squash and the bone broth into the pot. Bring to a simmer. Allow the mixture to simmer for about 5 minutes to let the flavors combine.

4. Turn off the heat and allow the soup to cool for a few minutes. Puree the soup in a blender or food processor. If necessary, do this in several batches; then return the soup to a clean pot. If the soup is too thick for your taste, add a little bit more bone broth. Season with a pinch or two of sea salt.

5. Garnish with cilantro and avocado and serve.

30-MINUTE KALE CHICKEN SOUP

Yield: 8 to 10 servings

Ingredients

3 tablespoons cultured ghee

2 cups sweet Vidalia or yellow onion (about 2 medium onions), peeled and diced small

1 cup celery (about 2 stalks), sliced thin

2 to 3 cups green cabbage (about ½ small head of cabbage), sliced into thin ribbons

4 garlic cloves, peeled and finely minced

8 cups homemade bone broth

3 to 4 cups cooked chicken, shredded (I use leftover chicken from making bone broth)

1 tablespoon dried parsley

1 teaspoon dried oregano

1 teaspoons sea salt, or to taste

1 teaspoon black pepper, or to taste

Leaves from 4 large stalks of kale, torn into bite-sized pieces (discard the center thick rib)

1 cup zucchini (about 1 medium zucchini), diced small

1 tablespoon lemon juice, optional

Directions

1. In a large Dutch oven or stockpot, combine the ghee, onion, and celery, and sauté over medium-high heat for about 7 minutes, or until the vegetables begin to soften. Stir intermittently.

2. Add the cabbage and sauté for about 3 minutes, or until the cabbage wilts and softens. Stir intermittently.

3. Add the garlic and sauté for another 1 to 2 minutes.

4. Add the bone broth, chicken, parsley, oregano, and salt and pepper to taste; and boil about 5 minutes, or until the chicken is warmed through.

5. Add the kale, zucchini, and lemon juice, and boil 1 to 2 minutes or until the kale has wilted and the zucchini has softened.

6. Taste the soup and add more salt, pepper, or herbs, to taste. At any time while making the soup, if the overall liquid level is lower than you like and you prefer more broth, add 1 or 2 cups of filtered water. Serve immediately. Soup will keep airtight in the fridge for 5 to 7 days or in the freezer for up to 6 months.

CHICKEN BONE BROTH

Yield: 14 to 16 servings

Ingredients

4 quarts cold, filtered water

2 tablespoons vinegar

1 large onion, coarsely chopped

2 carrots, peeled and coarsely chopped

3 celery stalks, coarsely chopped

1 whole free-range chicken or 2 to 3 pounds of bony chicken
   parts, such as necks, backs, breastbones, and wings*

Gizzards from one chicken (optional)

2 to 4 chicken feet

1 bunch parsley

*Note: Farm-raised, free-range chickens give the best results. Conventionally raised chickens will not produce stock that gels.

Directions

1. Fill a stockpot with the water, vinegar, onion, carrots, and celery. If you are using a whole chicken, put the whole chicken (removing the gizzard bag) in the stockpot; if you're using chicken pieces, put all of them in the stockpot. Add the gizzards and chicken feet. Let stand 60 minutes (this process helps break the bones down, so don't skip!).

2. Bring the pot to a boil, and remove scum that rises to the top. Reduce the heat, cover, and simmer for 8 to 12 hours. The longer you cook the stock, the richer and more flavorful it will be. However, longer-cooked stock also contains higher levels of histamines, which can be very inflammatory. So keep your cook time to 12 hours or less until the inflammation in your body is very low (you will be able to tell that inflammation is low when your red-flag symptoms subside).

3. About 10 minutes before finishing the stock, add parsley. This will impart additional mineral ions to the broth.

4. Let the soup cool down a bit until it's a little warmer than room temperature (or basically not too hot for you to get the chicken pieces out). Remove the whole chicken or chicken pieces with a slotted spoon, or strain the broth. You can reserve the chicken meat for other uses, such as chicken salads, enchiladas, sandwiches, or curries.

5. Strain the stock into a large bowl and reserve in your refrigerator and remove the congealed fat that rises to the top. Break the soup up into batches (I use 12-ounce mason jars) and freeze most of the broth immediately, leaving in the fridge only what you will consume over the next 2 to 3 days.

BEEF BONE BROTH

Yield: 14 to 16 servings

Ingredients

4 pounds beef marrow and knuckle bones
1 calf's foot (or 3 chicken feet), cut into pieces
½ cup vinegar
4 or more quarts cold, filtered water
3 pounds meaty rib or neck bones
3 onions, coarsely chopped
3 carrots, coarsely chopped

3 celery stalks, coarsely chopped
Several sprigs of fresh thyme, tied together
1 teaspoon dried green peppercorns, crushed
l bunch parsley

Directions

1. Preheat oven to 350 degrees.

2. Place the beef marrow and knuckle bones and the calf's foot in a very large pot with vinegar, and cover with water. Let stand for one hour.

3. Meanwhile, place the meaty bones in a roasting pan and brown in the oven. When it's well browned, add it to the pot, along with the onions, carrots, and celery.

4. Pour the fat out of the roasting pan, add some cold water to the pan, set over a high flame, and bring to a boil, stirring with a wooden spoon to loosen up coagulated juices. Add this liquid to the pot with the bones. Add additional water, if necessary, to cover the bones, but the liquid should come no higher than within 1 inch of the rim of the pot, as the volume expands slightly during cooking.

5. Bring the pot to a boil. A large amount of scum will come to the top, and it is important to remove it with a spoon. After you have skimmed the scum, reduce the heat and add the thyme and peppercorns.

6. Simmer the stock for 12 hours. The longer you cook the stock, the richer and more flavorful it will be. However, longer-cooked stock also contains higher levels of histamines, which can be very inflammatory. So keep your cook time to 12 hours or less until the inflammation in your body is very low (you will be able to tell that inflammation is low when your red-flag symptoms subside).

7. About 10 minutes before finishing the stock, add parsley. This will impart additional mineral ions to the broth. You will now have a pot of rather repulsive-looking brown liquid containing globs of gelatinous and fatty material. It won't even smell

particularly good. But don't fret—after straining it you will have a delicious and nourishing clear broth that is the ultimate tonic for lasting and thriving health.

8. Let the soup cool down to slightly warmer than room temperature. Remove the bones with tongs or a slotted spoon.

9. Strain the stock into a large bowl. Reserve in the refrigerator and remove the congealed fat that rises to the top. Break the soup into batches (I use 12-ounce mason jars) and freeze most of the broth immediately, leaving in the fridge only what you will consume over the next 2 to 3 days.

FISH BONE BROTH

Ideally, fish stock is made from the bones of sole or turbot. In Europe you can buy these fish on the bone. The fishmonger skins and filets the fish for you, giving you the filets for your evening meal and the bones for making the stock and final sauce. Unfortunately, in America sole arrives at the fish market preboned. But snapper, rockfish, and other non-oily fish work equally well, and good fish merchants will save the carcasses for you if you ask them. As they normally throw these carcasses away, they shouldn't charge you for them. Be sure to take the heads as well as the body—these are especially rich in iodine and fat-soluble vitamins. Classic cooking texts advise against using oily fish such as salmon for making broth, probably because highly unsaturated fish oils become rancid during the long cooking process.

Yield: 14 to 16 servings

Ingredients
2 tablespoons cultured ghee
2 onions, coarsely chopped
1 carrot, coarsely chopped

½ cup dry white wine or vermouth

3 or 4 whole carcasses, including heads, of non-oily fish such as sole, turbot, rockfish, or snapper

¼ cup vinegar

About 3 quarts cold, filtered water

Several sprigs fresh thyme

Several sprigs fresh parsley

1 bay leaf

Directions

1. Melt ghee in a large stainless steel pot. Add the onions and carrot, and cook them until they are soft, about a half hour.

2. Add the wine and bring to a boil.

3. Add the fish carcasses and cover with the cold, filtered water. Add vinegar. Bring to a boil and skim off the scum and impurities as they rise to the top.

4. Add the thyme, parsley, and bay leaf to the pot (you can tie them with twine or keep them loose). Reduce heat, cover, and simmer for 8 to 12 hours.

5. Remove carcasses with tongs or a slotted spoon, and strain the liquid into pint-sized storage containers. Reserve in the refrigerator and remove the congealed fat that rises to the top. Break the soup up into batches (I use 12-ounce mason jars) and freeze most of the broth immediately, leaving in the fridge only what you will consume over the next 2 to 3 days.

CROCK-POT BONE BROTH

I know not everyone likes to leave a cooking pot of bone broth on the stove for 12 hours, so there's another option: making broth in your crock-pot or Instant Pot.

Yield: 6 to 8 servings

Ingredients

1 to 2 pounds organic and grass-fed animal bones. (Chicken, beef, duck, bison, turkey, or lamb bones will work. Ask your local butcher for some bones if you don't have any left over.)

2 organic celery stalks, chopped in half

1 large organic carrot, chopped into chunks

1 medium onion, peeled and chopped in half

9 to 10 cups filtered water

Salt and pepper, to taste

Directions

1. Put the bones, celery, carrot, and onion into the slow-cooker and top with water until covered.

2. Cook on low for 12 hours. The longer you cook the stock, the richer and more flavorful it will be. However, longer-cooked stock also contains higher levels of histamines, which can be very inflammatory. So keep your cook time to 12 hours or less until the inflammation in your body is very low (you will be able to tell that inflammation is low when your red-flag symptoms subside).

3. After an hour or so, skim any "gunk" that is floating on the top.

4. Strain the broth into a bowl to separate the bones and vegetables from the liquid.

5. Season the broth with salt and pepper as desired.

6. Reserve in the refrigerator and remove the congealed fat that rises to the top. Break the soup up into batches (I use 12-ounce mason jars) and freeze most of the broth immediately, leaving in the fridge only what you will consume over the next 2 to 3 days.

INSTANT POT BONE BROTH

Yield: 10 to 12 servings

Ingredients

1 whole free-range chicken or 2 to 3 pounds of bony chicken
   parts, such as necks, backs, breastbones, and wings
Gizzards from one chicken (optional)
2 to 4 chicken feet
½ large onion, chopped
4 to 6 carrots, chopped
4 stalks celery, chopped
1 teaspoon apple cider vinegar
Filtered water
1 handful parsley, chopped

Directions

1. Place all ingredients except the filtered water and parsley in your Instant Pot.

2. Add filtered water until it's two-thirds full, or about 1 inch below the max line.

3. Let all the ingredients sit for 30 minutes in your Instant Pot; this allows the apple cider vinegar to break down the bones and collagen of the chicken parts.

4. Set Instant Pot to Soup, then manually change the time to 119 minutes.

5. After two hours, allow the Instant Pot to depressurize naturally.

6. Once you can open your Instant Pot, add parsley. Let it sit for about 20 minutes while the parsley helps pull even more nutrients from the bones.

7. Strain the broth and discard the bones and vegetables. Pour broth into jars, freezing most of it and storing some in the refrigerator to consume right away. I freeze mine in smaller batches, usually in 8- to 12-ounce containers, so that I can defrost as needed and the broth stays more fresh.

TURMERIC GINGER BONE BROTH

Yield: 10 to 12 servings

Ingredients

¼ teaspoon mustard seeds

2 teaspoon cumin seeds (or 1 teaspoon ground)

2 teaspoon coriander seeds (or 1 teaspoon ground)

2 tablespoons cultured ghee

1 onion, diced

1 piece lemongrass (remove outer hull, bruise the remaining layers with a knife, and chop finely)

1 ½ tablespoons ginger, finely chopped (or 2 teaspoons ground)

1 ½ tablespoons freshly grated turmeric (or 2 teaspoons ground)

4 garlic cloves, minced

4 cups filtered water

4 cups bone broth

1 teaspoon sea salt

2 teaspoons apple cider vinegar

A few sprigs of cilantro, for garnish

Scallions, chopped, for garnish

A few sprigs of mint, for garnish

1 avocado, diced, for garnish

Directions

1. Crush the mustard seeds, cumin seeds, and coriander seeds with a mortar and pestle (or spice grinder) as finely as possible. If using ground spices, then skip this step.

2. In a large, heavy-bottomed pot or Dutch oven, heat the ghee over medium-high heat.

3. Add the onion and sauté for 5 minutes. Add the lemongrass, ginger, and fresh turmeric and lower the heat to medium. Sauté for 5 minutes until it all starts to brown, stirring often.

4. Add the garlic and sauté for 2 more minutes.

5. Add the ground spices and sauté for 1 more minute.

6. Add the water, bone broth, and salt and bring to a simmer.

7. Add the apple cider vinegar.

8. Adjust your seasonings to taste. Garnish with cilantro, scallions, mint, and avocado.

9. Reserve in the refrigerator. Break the soup up into batches (I use 12-ounce mason jars) and freeze most of the broth immediately, leaving in the fridge only what you will consume over the next 2 to 3 days.

YOLKOCADO

Yield: 1 serving

Ingredients
1 avocado
2 separate egg yolks
Sea salt
Pepper

Directions

1. Preheat the oven to 425 degrees.

2. Slice the avocado in half, and take out the pit.

3. Place the avocado halves in a small baking dish.

4. Put an egg yolk into each avocado half.

5. Bake for 15 to 20 minutes.

6. Remove from the oven, and season with sea salt and pepper.

NO-MATO SAUCE

Adapted from Amanda Torres

Note: this recipe yields about 8 ½ cups sauce, so make a batch and freeze some of it for any time you want a marinara-like sauce. It's great over zoodles!

Yield: 4 to 5 servings

Ingredients

2 to 4 tablespoons of grass-fed ghee or coconut oil
4 to 8 cloves garlic, pressed or finely minced
4 ribs celery, chopped
1 large onion, chopped
3 medium beets, chopped
1 pound carrots, chopped
2 cups bone broth (less for a thicker sauce)
½ teaspoon dried basil
½ teaspoon dried oregano
½ teaspoon dried thyme
¼ teaspoon dried marjoram
2 dried bay leaves
Juice from 2 lemons
15 to 20 kalamata olives, pitted
Sea salt and pepper to taste

Directions

1. Heat the fat of choice in a large pot over medium-low heat for several minutes.

2. Add the garlic, celery, and onion to the pot and cook, stirring a few times, until the onion is translucent.

3. Add the beets and carrots and cook until soft, stirring a few times.

4. Add the broth, using just enough to cover the ingredients (or less for a thicker, less watery sauce).

5. Add the basil, oregano, thyme, marjoram, and bay leaves. Then add the lemon juice and stir well to combine everything. Bring to a boil, then reduce the heat to a simmer and cover. Simmer about 30 minutes, or until all the vegetables are tender. Stir about halfway through cooking.

6. Cool the sauce, remove the bay leaves, and blend in a blender. (Avoid putting a very hot sauce into a plastic blender, as chemicals will leach out into your food.)

7. Add the kalamata olives and salt and pepper to taste.

ZOODLES (A.K.A. ZUCCHINI NOODLES)

Zoodles are a great alternative to pasta, and a great way to increase your veggie intake. You will need a spiralizer to make them.

Yield: 2 to 4 servings

Ingredients
1 medium zucchini (for 2 servings)

Directions

1. Wash and trim the ends of the zucchini. And then spiralize! It's that simple. You can eat zoodles lightly steamed, or throw some into a cup of bone broth!

KALE CHIPS

Yield: 6 to 8 servings

Ingredients
2 cups fresh kale
1 tablespoon melted/liquefied ghee or coconut oil
1 tablespoon organic raw-coconut aminos (soy-free soy sauce)
Pinch of sea salt

Directions

1. Preheat oven to 350 degrees.

2. Remove all the hard stalks from the kale, then wash and allow the leaves to dry (you can pat them down with paper towels to speed up the drying process).

3. Tear kale into tortilla-chip-sized pieces.

4. Once the leaves are dry, place them in a large bowl and gently toss with the melted ghee, or coconut oil and the organic raw-coconut aminos.

5. Spread out evenly on an ungreased baking sheet. Sprinkle the kale with a pinch or two of sea salt.

6. Bake for 5 to 10 minutes, until the leaves are lightly brown near the edges and crispy.

CAULIFLOWER FRIED RICE

Yield: 4 to 6 servings

Ingredients

1 medium head of cauliflower
¼ cup coconut aminos
4 tablespoons ghee, melted
1 teaspoon ginger, minced
¼ teaspoon white pepper
2 egg yolks, beaten
3 garlic cloves, minced
1 medium onion, diced
½ cup broccoli florets
2 carrots, diced
3 scallions, chopped

Directions

1. Pulse the cauliflower in the bowl of a food processor until it resembles rice, about 2 to 3 minutes; set it aside.

2. In a small bowl, whisk together the coconut aminos, 2 tablespoons of melted ghee (or coconut oil), ginger and white pepper; set it aside.

3. Heat 1 tablespoon of ghee in a medium skillet over low heat. Add the beaten egg yolks and cook until cooked through (without mixing), about 2 to 3 minutes per side, flipping only once. Let cool before dicing into small pieces; set it aside.

4. Heat the remaining 1 tablespoon of ghee in a large skillet or wok over medium-high heat. Add the garlic and onion to the skillet, and cook, stirring often, until the onions have become translucent, about 3 to 4 minutes. Stir in the broccoli, carrots, and scallions. Cook, stirring constantly, until vegetables are tender, about 3 to 4 minutes.

5. Stir in the cauliflower, cooked eggs, and coconut aminos mixture. Cook, stirring constantly, until heated through and the cauliflower is tender, about 3 to 4 minutes. Serve immediately.

GUACAMOLE

Yield: 4 to 6 servings

Ingredients

1 small red onion, diced
2 cloves garlic, crushed with a garlic press
Juice from a whole lime
A handful of cilantro, chopped
Sea salt and pepper to taste
3 ripe avocados, pitted

Directions

1. Mix the onion and garlic in a medium mixing bowl.

2. Add lime juice, cilantro, sea salt, and pepper.

3. Add avocado and mash with a fork. Guacamole should have some lumps left; it should not be perfectly smooth.

CHOCOLATE COCONUT POWER BALLS

Adapted from UnboundWellness.com

Yield: 8 to 10 servings

Ingredients

1 cup coconut cream concentrate/coconut butter
¾ cup shredded coconut, plus extra for garnish
2 scoops Vital Proteins collagen powder
1 tablespoon coconut oil
1 tablespoon carob powder
2 tablespoons filtered water

Directions

1. Soften the coconut butter (leave it out at room temperature, or heat it in a saucepan just enough to soften it but not entirely melt it).

2. Fold in the remainder of the ingredients and stir well until evenly combined. Add more water if too thick.

3. Once combined, begin rolling the mixture into balls about ½-inch wide, or to the size of your liking, and sprinkle with extra shredded coconut for garnish.

4. Place in the refrigerator for at least 1 hour, or in the freezer if you plan to travel with them. Store the extras in the fridge.

PARSNIP CHIPS

Yield: 8 to 10 servings

Ingredients

4 tablespoons melted ghee or coconut oil
2 large parsnips, thinly sliced with mandoline slicer
¼ teaspoon sea salt

Directions

1. Preheat the oven to 350°F, and grease 2 baking sheets with 2 tablespoons of melted ghee or coconut oil.

2. In a large bowl, combine the parsnip slices, 2 tablespoons melted ghee or coconut oil, and sea salt. Toss until the parsnip slices are coated in fat and salt.

3. Place the parsnip slices onto greased baking sheets.

4. Cook for 6 to 8 minutes until golden brown.

PLANTAIN CHIPS

Yield: 4 to 6 servings

Ingredients

1 green plantain
1 teaspoon melted coconut oil
¼ teaspoon sea salt

Directions

1. Preheat the oven to 350°F, and line a baking sheet with unbleached parchment paper (it *must* be unbleached) or grease a baking sheet with ghee.

2. Cut the ends off the plantain and then score the length of it with about three evenly spaced cuts. Don't cut too far into the flesh; you want to cut just through the skin.

3. Peel the plantain and slice it on a diagonal as thinly as you can consistently manage.

4. Toss the plantain slices with the melted coconut oil, lay them out on the baking sheet, and sprinkle them with the salt.

5. Bake for 20 to 25 minutes or until golden brown.

AMAZING MAYONNAISE

Yield: 8 to 10 servings

Ingredients
2 egg yolks
1 teaspoon mustard (optional)
1 teaspoon horseradish (optional)
3 teaspoons lemon juice, divided
½ cup olive oil
½ cup coconut oil, melted
Sea salt
Pepper

Directions

1. In a blender or food processor, mix the yolks, mustard, horseradish, and 1 teaspoon of lemon juice.

2. In a separate bowl or mixing cup, whisk together the olive oil and coconut oil.

3. Set your blender or food processor to low and pour in the mixture of olive and coconut oil very slowly, even drop by drop in the beginning. You're creating an emulsion, and if you put too much oil in at once, the mixture will separate and be very hard to save.

4. As you add more oil, the emulsion will form and the mayonnaise will start to thicken, at which point you can pour the oil faster.

5. When all the oil is incorporated and the mayonnaise is thick, whisk in the rest of the lemon juice.

6. Season to taste with sea salt and pepper.

LIVER SUPPORT JUICE

Yield: 3 to 4 servings

Ingredients

4 beets, cooked

3 carrots, blanched

1-inch piece fresh ginger, peeled and minced

4 to 6 pieces of fresh turmeric (or 1 heaping teaspoon ground turmeric)

1 large handful of cilantro, stems included

1 large handful of dandelion greens, stems included

1 large handful of parsley

Juice of 2 lemons

¼ teaspoon freshly ground black pepper

¼ teaspoon sea salt

1 garlic clove (or ¼ teaspoon organic garlic powder for a milder flavor)

Directions

1. Blend all the ingredients; add ½ cup of filtered water if it's too thick for your liking. Enjoy! Makes 2 to 3 servings. Reserve additional servings, broken up into 8-ounce portions in the freezer, and thaw as needed.

GINGER TEA

Yield: 4 servings

Ingredients

4 cups water
4-inch piece of fresh ginger root, peeled and diced
Lemon slices or the juice of a full lemon, to taste

Directions

1. Bring the water to a full boil.

2. Add the ginger to the boiling water and reduce to simmer for 8 to 10 minutes.

3. Remove the pot from the stove. Strain the tea into a cup through a fine-mesh strainer to filter out the particles of turmeric and ginger. Add lemon to taste.

4. Serve hot as tea during the winter or cool as a lemonade in summer.

THE PURIFY SMOOTHIE

Yield: 1 serving

Ingredients

1 cup coconut yogurt (either homemade or the brand Anita's) or 1 cup full-fat coconut milk (I like the brands Native Forest and Let's Do Organic)
1 cup filtered water, plus more to taste
½ avocado
1 scoop of bone broth protein (I like the Dr. Axe brand)
1 scoop of collagen peptides (I like the Vital Proteins brand)
¼ teaspoon cinnamon

1 teaspoon turmeric
1 teaspoon ground ginger
2 cups blanched spinach or kale
¼ teaspoon ground Himalayan sea salt

Directions

1. Blend all the ingredients. Add another ½ cup filtered water if it's too thick for your liking. Enjoy!

ULTIMATE PREBIOTIC SALAD

Yield: 2 to 3 servings

Ingredients

Salad:
2 cups kale, finely sliced
2 cups dandelion greens, finely sliced
Juice of ½ lemon
1 carrot, grated
1 leek, sliced thinly, white part only
¼-inch ginger root, peeled and minced
1 small red onion, sliced thinly
5 stalks of steamed asparagus, diced
2 to 3 Jerusalem artichokes, sliced thinly
2 to 3 radishes, sliced thinly
1 avocado, diced
Spoonful of sauerkraut (optional)

Garlic dressing:
2 cloves garlic, finely chopped
1 tablespoon sea salt
2 tablespoons lemon juice
¼ cup balsamic vinegar
¼ cup virgin olive oil

Directions

1. Massage the kale and dandelion greens with the lemon juice in a large salad bowl and leave to wilt for 10 to 20 minutes.

2. Add the carrot, leek, ginger, onion, asparagus, artichokes, radishes, and avocado, and toss. Top with the sauerkraut.

3. Make the dressing. Mix the garlic with the salt, and mash them together using either the back of a knife or a mortar and pestle, to make a paste. Transfer to a small bowl. Add the lemon juice and balsamic vinegar. Gradually whisk in the olive oil. Taste for tartness and adjust. If you need to make it milder, add more olive oil.

4. Pour the dressing over the salad until well combined.

MAGNESIUM OIL SPRAY

Yield: 300 servings/sprays (1 cup or 8 ounces total)

Ingredients
½ cup distilled water
½ cup magnesium-chloride flakes (I like the brand Ancient Minerals)

Directions

1. Boil the distilled water. It is important to use distilled water to extend the shelf life of the mixture.

2. Place the magnesium-chloride flakes in a glass bowl or measuring cup, and then pour the boiling water over it.

3. Stir well until completely dissolved. Let cool completely and store in a glass spray bottle. The spray can be stored at room temperature for at least 6 months.

On-the-Go
Snack Ideas

I know how hectic life can be, so I went ahead and gathered a list of easy on-the-go snacks that can be store-bought. As of January 2017, these snacks and brands are all *Body Belief*–approved, but always read the ingredients to be certain:

EPIC Bison Bacon Cranberry Bar
Organic Gemini TigerNut Raw Snack
Artisana Organics Raw Coconut Butter
Bare Organic Cinnamon Apple Chips
Dang Coconut Chips
Nutiva Coconut Manna
Jackson's Honest Sweet Potato Chips
Natierra Nature's All Foods Freeze-Dried Blueberries
SeaSnax Roasted Seaweed
Wild Planet Wild Pink Salmon, Alaskan
Wild Planet Wild Sardines
Eden Foods Apple Butter, Organic
Pork Clouds Fried Pork Rinds, Rosemary & Sea Salt
Paleo Angel Power Balls (or make your own!)
Mission Heirloom Yucan Crunch
Wild Zora Mediterranean Lamb Bars with Spinach, Rosemary
    & Turmeric
Pure Traditions Mountain Strips—Cranberry (beef and organ
    power snacks)
Inka Crops Plantain Chips
Anita's Coconut Milk Yogurt Alternative, Plain
GT's Kombucha

Keep in mind you will likely be able to find all these products online.

Body Belief–Approved Personal-Care Products

These are solely products that meet my standard of recommendation, and that I encourage you to try as you reawaken your health. I am not receiving any compensation for recommending any of the products listed below, except the ones made by me and sold on AimeeRauppBeauty.com, as noted. As of January 2017, all products scored a 2 or lower on the Environmental Working Group's cosmetic-database site (www.ewg.org) and the Think Dirty product-evaluation site (www.thinkdirtyapp.com). But please continue to check the scores of all products, since formulations can change, and therefore toxicity levels can change too.

Body Lotion

- Aimee Raupp Beauty Organic Body Butter | aimeerauppbeauty.com
- 100% PURE Nourishing Body Cream | www.100percentpure.com
- Wildly Organic Cold-Pressed Coconut Oil, Virgin Unrefined | wildernessfamilynaturals.com
- Nubian Heritage Raw Shea Butter Body Lotion| www.nubianheritage.com
- The Honest Company Face + Body Lotion | www.honest.com

Shampoo

- Primal Life Organics Shampoo Bar or Dirty Poo Hair Wash | www.primallifeorganics.com
- ACURE Organics (various) | www.acureorganics.com
- Dr. Ron's MSM shampoos | www.drrons.com
- The Honest Company Shampoo + Body Wash | www.honest.com
- Kiss My Face Big Body Shampoo | kissmyface.com

Soap/Body Wash

- Primal Life Organics Dirty Body Bar | www.primallifeorganics.com
- The Honest Company Shampoo + Body Wash | www.honest.com
- ACURE Organics body wash | www.acureorganics.com
- Aveeno Moisturizing Bar | www.aveeno.com
- Dr. Bronner's Pure Castile Soap | drbronner.com

Face Wash

- Aimee Raupp Beauty Argan Oil Facial Cleanser | aimeerauppbeauty.com
- Primal Life Organics face washes | www.primallifeorganics.com
- ACURE Organics facial cleansers | www.acureorganics.com

- 100% PURE facial cleansers|
  www.100percentpure.com
- Neutrogena Ultra Gentle Hydrating Cleanser | www.
  neutrogena.com

Facial Scrub

- Aimee Raupp Beauty Organic Coconut Sugar Facial
  Scrub | aimeerauppbeauty.com
- Primal Life Organics Dirty Ex Sweet Revenge Face
  Exfoliator | www.primallifeorganics.com
- suki Exfoliate Foaming Cleanser | sukiskincare.com

Facial Moisturizer

- Aimee Raupp Beauty Organic Balancing Facial Oil |
  aimeerauppbeauty.com
- Primal Life Organics Bare Face Moisturizer | www.
  primallifeorganics.com
- 100% PURE facial moisturizers |
  www.100percentpure.com
- ACURE Organics Day Cream | www.
  acureorganics.com
- The Honest Company Face + Body Lotion | www.
  honest.com

Toner

- Aimee Raupp Beauty Organic Rose Facial Toner | aimeerauppbeauty.com
- Just the Goods Vegan Facial Toner | justthegoods.net
- Primal Life Organics toners (multiple formulas) | www.primallifeorganics.com
- White & Elm Balancing Facial Toner | www.whiteandelm.com

Eye Cream

- Aimee Raupp Beauty Organic Cocoa Butter Eye Cream | aimeerauppbeauty.com
- goop by Juice Beauty Perfecting Eye Cream | shop.goop.com
- 100% PURE Coffee Bean Caffeine Eye Cream | www.100percentpure.com
- Herbal Choice Mari Organic Eye Cream | www.naturesbrands.com

Blemish Treatment

- Aimee Raupp Beauty Organic Blemish-Be-Gone Stick | aimeerauppbeauty.com
- Primal Life Organics Banished Blemish Serum | www.primallifeorganics.com
- Herbal Choice Mari Facial Blemish Treatment | www.naturesbrands.com
- Organic tea tree essential oil | multiple retailers

Deodorant

- Primal Life Organics Stick Up | www.primallife organics.com
- Tom's of Maine Mineral Confidence Deodorant Crystal | www.tomsofmaine.com
- Crystal Body Deodorant | www.thecrystal.com
- Thai Crystal Deodorant | www.iherb.com

Lip Balm

- Aimee Raupp Beauty Organic Lip Butter | aimeerauppbeauty.com
- Primal Life Organics Grunt Lip Balm | www.primallifeorganics.com
- Badger's Classic Unscented Lip Balm | www.badgerbalm.com
- Beautycounter Lip Conditioner | www.beautycounter.com
- eos Lip Balm | evolutionofsmooth.com

Lipstick/Lip Gloss

- Aimee Raupp Beauty Organic Tinted Lip Butter: Rose Cinnamon | aimeerauppbeauty.com
- Modern Minerals Emotive or Invigorating Lip Gloss | modernmineralsmakeup.com
- Beautycounter Lip Gloss | www.beautycounter.com

- Au Naturale Cosmetics lipsticks |
  www.aunaturalecosmetics.com
- Sally B's B Glossy Lip Gloss |
  www.sallybskinyummies.com

Foundation/Tinted Moisturizer

- Modern Minerals powder foundation |
  modernmineralsmakeup.com
- Primal Life Organics foundations |
  www.primallifeorganics.com
- W3LL PEOPLE Narcissist Foundation Stick |
  w3llpeople.com
- 100% PURE Fruit Pigmented Healthy Foundation |
  www.100percentpure.com

Eye Shadow

- Modern Minerals eye shadows |
  modernmineralsmakeup.com
- Primal Life Organics Lid Stains |
  www.primallifeorganics.com
- e.l.f. Cosmetics Mad for Matte Eyeshadow |
  www.elfcosmetics.com
- Au Naturale eye shadow |
  www.aunaturalecosmetics.com

Mascara

- W3LL PEOPLE Expressionist Mascara | w3llpeople.com
- Physicians Formula Organic wear 100% Natural Origin Mascara | www.physiciansformula.com
- 100% PURE mascaras | www.100percentpure.com
- Beautycounter Lengthening Mascara | www.beautycounter.com
- e.l.f. Cosmetics Mineral Infused Mascara | www.elfcosmetics.com

Nail Polish

- Pacifica nail polishes | www.pacificabeauty.com
- Smith & Cult Color | www.smithandcult.com
- butter LONDON nail lacquers | www.butterlondon.com
- Deborah Lippmann nail polish | www.deborahlippmann.com
- Julep nail polish | www.julep.com

Body Belief–Approved Household and Cleaning Products

The best way to clean your home is to use basic nontoxic ingredients like your grandmother used. Here's a breakdown of some of these substances and what they're good for:

Baking Soda—cleans, deodorizes, softens water, and scours.

Lemon—one of the strongest food acids, effective against most household bacteria.

Borax (sodium borate)—cleans; deodorizes; disinfects; softens water; cleans wallpaper, painted walls, and floors.

White Vinegar—cuts grease; removes mildew, odors, some stains, and wax build-up.

Washing Soda (a.k.a. sal soda or sodium carbonate decahydrate)—cuts grease; removes stains; softens water; cleans wall, tiles, sinks, and tubs. Use care, as washing soda can irritate mucous membranes. Do not use on aluminum.

Cornstarch—cleans windows, polishes furniture, shampoos carpets and rugs.

Citrus Solvent—cleans paintbrushes, oil and grease, and some stains. Use care, as citrus solvent may cause skin, lung, or eye irritations for people with multiple chemical sensitivities.

With these ingredients in mind, here are some great DIY house-cleaning formulations to safely clean your home:

All-Purpose Cleaner: Mix ½ cup vinegar and ¼ cup baking soda (or 2 teaspoons borax) into ½ gallon (2 liters) water. Store and keep. Use for removal of water-deposit stains on shower-stall panels, bathroom chrome fixtures, windows, bathroom mirrors, etc.

Dishwasher Soap: Mix equal parts of borax and washing soda (increase the washing soda if your water is hard.)

Disinfectant: Mix 2 teaspoons borax, 4 tablespoons vinegar, and 3 cups hot water. For stronger cleaning power, add ¼ teaspoon liquid castile soap like Dr. Bronner's. Wipe on with dampened cloth or use a nonaerosol spray bottle. (This is not an antibacterial formula. The average kitchen or bathroom does not require antibacterial cleaners.)

Furniture Polish: Mix equal parts olive oil and lemon juice.

Mold Remover: Mix 1 part tea tree essential oil to 5 parts water. For those of you who want to purchase commercial nontoxic cleaning products, here are some of my favorites (but keep in mind, just as with makeup and skincare, these formulations can change and become more toxic, so always read ingredients and avoid the 15 toxic ingredients I discussed on pp. 130–133):

Dishwasher Soap: Nellie's All-Natural Automatic Dishwasher Powder, Earth Friendly Wave Auto Dishwasher Gel, GreenShield Organic Automatic Dishwasher Liquid Gel, MamaSuds Automatic Dishwasher Powder, The Honest Company Auto Dishwasher Gel.

Dish Soap: Dr. Bronner's Pure-Castile Soap, CitraDish Natural Dish Soap, Ecover Dish Soap (unscented), MamaSuds Castile Soap, The Honest Company Dish Soap

Multipurpose Cleaner: CitraSolv Plant-Based Multi-Purpose Cleaner, Babyganics Multi Surface Cleaner, AspenClean All Purpose Cleaner, BioKleen All Purpose Cleaner, Dr. Bronner's Sal Suds Biodegradable Cleaner, Whole Foods Market Organic All-Purpose Spray

Laundry Detergent: Nellie's All-Natural Laundry Soda, CitraSuds Natural Laundry Detergent, Eco Nuts Organic Laundry Detergent Soap Nuts, Whole Foods Market Organic Laundry Detergent (unscented)

For more nontoxic household cleaning products, visit Environmental Working Group's guide to healthy cleaning (http://www.ewg.org/guides/cleaners).

Conversion Charts

Standard Cup	Fine Powder (e.g., flour)	Grain (e.g., rice)	Granular (e.g., sugar)	Liquid Solids (e.g., butter)	Liquid (e.g., milk)
1	140 g	150 g	190 g	200 g	240 ml
¾	105 g	113 g	143 g	150 g	180 ml
⅔	93 g	100 g	125 g	133 g	160 ml
½	70 g	75 g	95 g	100 g	120 ml
⅓	47 g	50 g	63 g	67 g	80 ml
¼	35 g	38 g	48 g	50 g	60 ml
⅛	18 g	19 g	24 g	25 g	30 ml

Useful Equivalents for Liquid Ingredients by Volume				
¼ tsp				1 ml
½ tsp				2 ml
1 tsp				5 ml
3 tsp	1 tbsp		½ fl oz	15 ml
	2 tbsp	⅛ cup	1 fl oz	30 ml
	4 tbsp	¼ cup	2 fl oz	60 ml
	5⅓ tbsp	⅓ cup	3 fl oz	80 ml
	8 tbsp	½ cup	4 fl oz	120 ml
	10⅔ tbsp	⅔ cup	5 fl oz	160 ml
	12 tbsp	¾ cup	6 fl oz	180 ml
	16 tbsp	1 cup	8 fl oz	240 ml
	1 pt	2 cups	16 fl oz	480 ml
	1 qt	4 cups	32 fl oz	960 ml
			33 fl oz	1000 ml 1 liter

Useful Equivalents for Dry Ingredients by Weight

(To convert ounces to grams, multiply the number of ounces by 30.)

1 oz	¹⁄₁₆ lb	30 g
4 oz	¼ lb	120 g
8 oz	½ lb	240 g
12 oz	¾ lb	360 g
16 oz	1 lb	480 g

Useful Equivalents for Cooking/Oven Temperatures

Process	Fahrenheit	Celsius	Gas Mark
Freeze Water	32° F	0° C	
Room Temperature	68° F	20° C	
Boil Water	212° F	100° C	
Bake	325° F	160° C	3
	350° F	180° C	4
	375° F	190° C	5
	400° F	200° C	6
	425° F	220° C	7
	450° F	230° C	8
Broil			Grill

Useful Equivalents for Length

(To convert inches to centimeters, multiply the number of inches by 2.5.)

1 in			2.5 cm	
6 in	½ ft		15 cm	
12 in	1 ft		30 cm	
36 in	3 ft	1 yd	90 cm	
40 in			100 cm	1 m

Endnotes

Introduction

1. "What Thoughts and Emotions Are Affecting Your Cells? Here Is the Science Behind It," *The Biology of Belief* (blog), August 28, 2014, https://biologyofbelief.wordpress.com/2014/08/28/what-thoughts-and-emotions -are-affecting-your-cells-here-is-the-science-behind-it.

Chapter 1

1. Sarah Ballantyne, *The Paleo Approach: Reverse Autoimmune Disease and Heal Your Body* (New York: Victory Belt Publishing, 2013).

2. Donna Jackson Nakazawa, "The Autoimmune Epidemic: Bodies Gone Haywire in a World Out of Balance," *Alternet*, March 18, 2008, http://www .alternet.org/story/80129/the_autoimmune_epidemic%3A_bodies_gone_ haywire_in_a_world_out_of_balance.

3. Jeroen Visser et al., "Tight Junctions, Intestinal Permeability, and Autoimmunity Celiac Disease and Type 1 Diabetes Paradigms," *Annals of the New York Academy of Sciences* 1165 (2009): 195.

4. Ballantyne, *The Paleo Approach*.

5. Charles W. Schmidt, "Questions Persist: Environmental Factors in Autoimmune Disease," *Environmental Health Perspectives* 119, no. 6 (2011). https://www.ncbi.nlm.nih.gov/pmc/articles/PMC3114837.

6. Grace Rattue, "Autoimmune Disease Rates Increasing," *MedicalNewsToday*, June 22, 2012, http://www.medicalnewstoday.com/articles/246960.php.

7. Ron Breazeale, Ph.D., "Thoughts, Neurotransmitters, Body-Mind Connection," *Psychology Today*, July 7, 2012, https://www.psychology today.com/blog/in-the-face-adversity/201207/thoughts-neurotransmitters -body-mind-connection.

8. "What Thoughts and Emotions Are Affecting Your Cells?", *The Biology of Belief* (blog).

9. G. Vighi et al., "Allergy and the Gastrointestinal System," *Clinical & Experimental Immunology* (September 2008). https://www.ncbi.nlm.nih.gov /pmc/articles/PMC2515351.

10. Alessio Fasano and Terez Shea-Donohue, "Mechanisms of Disease: The Role of Intestinal Barrier Function in the Pathogenesis of Gastrointestinal Autoimmune Diseases," *Nature Reviews Gastroenterology & Hepatology* 2 (September 2005): 416–422. http://www.nature.com/nrgastro/journal/v2/n9 /full/ncpgasthep0259.html.

11. Alessio Fasano, "Leaky Gut and Autoimmune Diseases," *Clinical Reviews in Allergy & Immunology* 42 (February 2012): 71–8. https://www.ncbi.nlm.nih .gov/pubmed/22109896.

12. Alessio Fasano, "Zonulin, Regulation of Tight Junctions, and Autoimmune Diseases," *Annals of the New York Academy of Sciences* (July 2012): 25–33. https://www.ncbi.nlm.nih.gov/pubmed/22731712.

13. Visser, "Tight Junctions."

14. Frederick W. Miller et al., "Epidemiology of Environmental Exposures and Human Autoimmune Diseases: Findings from a National Institute of Environmental Health Sciences Expert Panel Workshop," Journal of Autoimmunity 39, no. 4 (December 2012): 259–271. https://www.ncbi.nlm .nih.gov/pmc/articles/PMC3496812.

15. Subhuti Dharmananda, Ph.D., "Autoimmune Diseases and the Potential Role of Chinese Herbal Medicine," Institute of Traditional Medicine, accessed 1/20/17, http://www.itmonline.org/arts/autoimmune.html.

Chapter 2

1. Barron H. Lerner, M.D., "When Med Students Get Medical Students' Disease," Well blog), *New York Times*, September 5, 2013, https://well.blogs.nytimes .com/2013/09/05/when-med-students-get-medical-students-disease/?_r=0.

2. Xiaosi Gu et al., "Belief about Nicotine Selectively Modulates Value and Reward Prediction Error Signals in Smokers," *Proceedings of the National Academy of Sciences of the United States of America* 112, no. 8 (February 24, 2015): 2539–2544. http://www.pnas.org/content/112/8/2539.

3. "Medical Definition of Placebo Effect," *MedicineNet,* accessed 1/20/2017, http://www.medicinenet.com/script/main/art.asp?articlekey=31481.

4. "Why Do Placebos Work?," *CBSNews.com*, October 9, 2016, https://www .cbsnews.com/news/why-do-placebos-work.

5. Candace B. Pert, Ph.D., *Everything You Need to Know to Feel Go(o)d* (Carlsbad, CA: Hay House, Inc., 2007), Kindle edition, 110.

6. Russ Gerber, "Belief and Its Effect on Our Health," *Psychology Today*, December 29, 2013, https://www.psychologytoday.com/blog/our-health /201312/belief-and-its-effect-our-health.

7. Sarah Rimer and Madeline Drexler, "The Biology of Emotion—and What It May Teach Us about Helping People to Live Longer," *Harvard Public Health*, Winter 2011, https://www.hsph.harvard.edu/news/magazine/happiness -stress-heart-disease.

8. Edward Diener and Micaela Y. Chan, "Happy People Live Longer: Subjective Well-Being Contributes to Health and Longevity," *Applied Psychology: Health and Well-Being* 3: 1–43. http://onlinelibrary.wiley.com/doi/10.1111/j.1758 -0854.2010.01045.x/abstract.

9. "The Health Benefits of Strong Relationships," Harvard Health Publishing, December 2010, accessed 1/20/2017, https://www.health.harvard.edu /newsletter_article/the-health-benefits-of-strong-relationships.

Chapter 4

1. Emma M Seppalla, Ph.D., "20 Scientific Reasons to Start Meditating Today," *Psychology Today*, September 11, 2013, https://www.psychologytoday.com /blog/feeling-it/201309/20-scientific-reasons-start-meditating-today.

Chapter 5

1. V. Michopoulos et al., "Inflammation in Fear- and Anxiety-Based Disorders: PTSD, GAD, and Beyond," *Neuropsychopharmacology* 42 (January 2017): 254–270. https://www.ncbi.nlm.nih.gov/pubmed/27510423.

Chapter 6

1. Visser, "Tight Junctions."

Chapter 7

1. Fasano, "Leaky Gut and Autoimmune Diseases."

2. Amy Myers, M.D., *The Autoimmune Solution: Prevent and Reverse the Full Spectrum of Inflammatory Symptoms and Diseases* (New York: HarperOne, 2017).

3. "The Downside of Soybean Consumption," *Nutrition Digest* 38, no. 2 (October 14, 2001), http://americannutritionassociation.org/newsletter /downside-soybean-consumption-0.

4. A. Bandyopadhyay, S. Ghoshal, and A. Mukherjee, "Genotoxicity Testing of Low-Calorie Sweeteners: Aspartame, Acesulfame-K, and Saccharin," *Drug and Chemical Toxicology* 31, no. 4 (2008): 447–57. https://www.ncbi.nlm.nih.gov/pubmed/18850355.

5. C. R. Whitehouse, J. Boullata, and L. A. McCauley, "The Potential Toxicity of Artificial Sweeteners, *AAOHN Journal* 56, no. 6 (June 2008): 251–9. https://www.ncbi.nlm.nih.gov/pubmed/18604921.

6. Richard P. Bazinet, Ph.D., and Michael W.A. Chu, M.D., M.Ed., "Omega-6 Polyunsaturated Fatty Acids: Is a Broad Cholesterol-Lowering Health Claim Appropriate?," *CMAJ* (November 11, 2013), http://www.cmaj.ca/content/early/2013/11/11/cmaj.130253.

7. E. Patterson et al., "Health Implications of High Dietary Omega-6 Polyunsaturated Fatty Acids," *Journal of Nutrition and Metabolism* (April 5, 2012). https://www.ncbi.nlm.nih.gov/pmc/articles/PMC3335257.

8. T. L. Blasbalq et al., "Changes in Consumption of Omega-3 and Omega-6 Fatty Acids in the United States During the 20th Century," *American Journal of Clinical Nutrition* 93, no. 5 (May 2011): 950–62. https://www.ncbi.nlm.nih.gov/pubmed/21367944.

9. Ballantyne, *The Paleo Approach*.

10. G. Francis et al., "The Biological Action of Saponins in Animal Systems: A Review," *British Journal of Nutrition* 88, no. 6 (December 2002): 587–605. https://www.ncbi.nlm.nih.gov/pubmed/12493081.

11. E. Jensen-Jarolim et al., "Hot Spices Influence Permeability of Human Intestinal Epithelial Monolayers," *Journal of Nutrition* 128, no. 3 (March 1998): 577–81. https://nova3labs.com/hot-peppers-gi-permeability.

12. Loren Cordain, Ph.D., "Egg Whites and Autoimmune Disease," *The Paleo Diet* (August 2015), http://thepaleodiet.com/wp-content/uploads/2015/08/Paleo-Paper-eggwhite.pdf.

Chapter 9

1. Michelle Persad, "The Average Woman Puts 515 Synthetic Chemicals on Her Body Every Day without Knowing," *HuffPost*, last modified March 7, 2016, http://www.huffingtonpost.com/entry/synthetic-chemicals-skincare_us_56d8ad09e4b0000de403d995.

2. Visser, "Tight Junctions."

3. Samim Ozen and Sukran Darcan, "Effects of Environmental Endocrine Disruptors on Pubertal Development," *Journal of Clinical Research in Pediatric Endocrinology* 3, no. 1 (March 2011): 1–6. https://www.ncbi.nlm.nih.gov/pmc/articles/PMC3065309.

Endnotes

4. A. Karwacka et al., "Exposure to Modern, Widespread Environmental Endocrine Disrupting Chemicals and Their Effect on the Reproductive Potential of Women: An Overview of Current Epidemiological Evidence," *Human Fertility* (July 31, 2017): 1–24. https://www.ncbi.nlm.nih.gov/pubmed/28758506.

5. H. J. Jang, C. Y. Shin, and K. B. Kim, "Safety Evaluation of Polyethylene Glycol (PEG) Compounds for Cosmetic Use," *Toxicological Research* 31, no. 2 (June 2015): 105–36. https://www.ncbi.nlm.nih.gov/pubmed/26191379.

6. "Formaldehyde and Cancer Risk." National Cancer Institute. https://www.cancer.gov/about-cancer/causes-prevention/risk/substances/formaldehyde/formaldehyde-fact-sheet.

7. Diane Taylor, "Take a Toxic Tour of Your Bathroom," *The Guardian*, February 25, 2003, U.S. edition, Health and Wellbeing section, https://www.theguardian.com/lifeandstyle/2003/feb/25/healthandwellbeing.health2.

8. A. M. Bougea et al., "Effect of the Emotional Freedom Technique on Perceived Stress, Quality of Life, and Cortisol Salivary Levels in Tension-type Headache Sufferers: A Randomized Controlled Trial," *Explore (N.Y.)* 9, no. 2 (March-April 2013): 91–9. https://www.ncbi.nlm.nih.gov/pubmed/23452711.

9. F. Liang et al., "Acupuncture and Immunity," *Evidence-Based Complementary and Alternative Medicine* (2015), https://www.hindawi.com/journals/ecam/2015/260620.

10. Sen Hu et al., "Electroacupuncture at Zusanli (ST36) Prevents Intestinal Barrier and Remote Organ Dysfunction Following Gut Ischemia through Activating the Cholinergic Anti-Inflammatory-Dependent Mechanism," *Evidence-Based Complementary and Alternative Medicine* (April 4, 2013), https://www.ncbi.nlm.nih.gov/pmc/articles/PMC3638586.

11. Z. Cho et al., "Neural Substrates, Experimental Evidences and Functional Hypothesis of Acupuncture Mechanisms," *Acta Neurologica Scandinavica* 113 (2006): 370–377. https://www.ncbi.nlm.nih.gov/pmc/articles/PMC3638586.

12. Dawson Church, Ph.D., Garret Yount, Ph.D., and Audrey J. Brooks, Ph.D., "The Effect of Emotional Freedom Techniques on Stress Biochemistry: A Randomized Controlled Trial," *Journal of Nervous and Mental Disease* 200, no. 10 (October 2012): 891–6. https://www.ncbi.nlm.nih.gov/pubmed/22986277.

Acknowledgments

This book wouldn't exist without my patients. Thank you to all of you—you are my greatest teachers and I am honored to share the path to wellness with you.

To my husband, Ken—you are my true love. Together we are the best versions of ourselves. Thank you for all of it and especially for our delicious family sandwiches.

To my sweet baby, Jaymes—you are my sunshine, my dearest sunshine, you take my happy to a whole new level. Forever.

To my mommy and daddy—from your love I was created and from that love comes the love I spread to millions. Thank you for all you give me. Every day I shine for you.

To my brother love, Harry, and my sister, Lily, and my love-bugs Sam and Ryan—I love you and I am honored to call you my family and my friends.

To my family: Uncle Eddie, Uncle Jim (in heaven), Blaguna, Uncle Mike, Aunt Dawn, Uncle Tom, and Uncle Monroe—you have always supported me and believed in me in the most beautiful ways. . . . I am so incredibly grateful for you all.

To the amazing new family members I happily (and luckily) acquired through marriage—Nancy, Christy, Andy, Bill, Donna, Aunt Barbara, Kaleigh, Ryan, Colin, and Annie—I love being a part of your family! Thank you for all your love and encouragement!

To my posse of likeminded friends: Melanie Vangopoulos, Nathalie Brochu, Hima Katari, Arielle Haspel, Gabby Bernstein, Agapi Stassinopoulos, Claudia Chan, Reshma Saujani, Brooke Thorburn, Heather Kreutter, Javi Ruiz, Jolie and Gabe Schwartz, Danielle Quintana, Johanna Berry-Wasser, Kimmy Holmstrom, Jessica Diamond-Meincke, Siobhan Carpenter, Athena Still, Kymberly Kelly, Sarah Coles McKeown, Katie Chatzopoulos, Ali Johnson, Sasha Weiss, Piper Weiss, Nicole Jardim, Rebecca Parekh—my appreciation for you is enormous. Thank you for sharing this journey with me, for supporting me and for always inspiring me.

To Sloane Miller—You rock! Thank you! Seriously . . . you're amazing and you help make book writing FUN!

To Anne Bohner—It's so uplifting and exciting working with you! Cheers to this project and many more! Thank you for always having my back.

To Richelle Fredson, Patty Gift, and the Hay House Team— your wisdom and insight helped bring this book to fruition. Thank you for believing in my mission.

To my amazing team: Jen Walters Burke and Beth Grossmann— you two are such an incredible part of my mission, spreading the message of reawakened health and wellness. I love you and I couldn't do any of this without you.

To all of those who have come to me for guidance, direction, and healing and to those of you who have guided, healed, and taught me—without you, none of this would be possible. Thank you for sharing your life with me. My world is a better place for having each of you in it.

To the love, light, and guidance that surrounds me each and every day—thank you for always having my back and encouraging me to continuously find joy and love in all that comes my way.

To my spiritual teachers who guide and inspire me to share the messages herein, your teachings have transformed my life and the lives of so many: Abraham Hicks, Wayne Dyer, Neville Goddard, Deepak Chopra and Gabrielle Bernstein and Louise Hay.

Damn, this is a good life, and I look forward to more, more, more!!!

Your *Body Belief* Guide

Heal yourself from autoimmune disease by reconnecting to yourself, renewing your beliefs, and ultimately reawakening your health. Join Aimee Raupp at www.aimeeraupp.com/bodybelief for numerous resources and tools to help you easily implement the Body Belief plan into your daily routine and start feeling your best. With her guidance, you will be on the path to shifting your health, healing from autoimmunity, and loving your body more. The Body Belief resources include:

1. **Free recipes, meal plans, and shopping lists—**
   everything you need to jump-start the Body Belief
   action plan

2. **Access to the Body Belief online support group—**
   join Aimee's private Facebook group to receive
   support from a community of women who are
   currently on the Body Belief plan and to have
   your questions answered directly by Aimee during
   regularly scheduled "office hours"

3. **Autoimmune yoga, EFT (Emotional Freedom
   Technique or tapping), and qi gong videos—**check
   out these mind-body tools to help you release stress
   and emotional blockages

By following the Body Belief lifestyle roadmap, your health will begin to thrive, both inside and out. To receive support on the healing journey, visit www.aimeeraupp.com/bodybelief. For thousands of recipes that fit into the Body Belief eating plan, head over to aimeeraupp.com/realplans.

About the Author

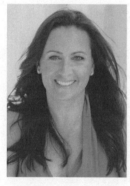

Aimee E. Raupp, M.S., L.Ac., is a renowned women's health-and-wellness expert and author. A licensed acupuncturist and herbalist in private practice in New York, Aimee holds a M.S. in Traditional Oriental Medicine from the Pacific College of Oriental Medicine and a B.A. in biology from Rutgers University. Aimee is also the founder of the Aimee Raupp Beauty line of hand-crafted, organic skincare products, a women's health expert, and an active contributor and columnist for many publications. You can visit her online at www.aimeeraupp.com.

Hay House Titles of Related Interest

YOU CAN HEAL YOUR LIFE, the movie,
starring Louise Hay & Friends
(available as a 1-DVD program, an expanded 2-DVD set,
and an online streaming video)
Learn more at www.hayhouse.com/louise-movie

THE SHIFT, the movie,
starring Dr. Wayne W. Dyer
available as a 1-DVD program, an expanded 2-DVD set,
and an online streaming video)
Learn more at www.hayhouse.com/the-shift-movie

———

*CULTURED FOOD IN A JAR: 100+ Probiotic Recipes to
Inspire and Change Your Life,* by Donna Schwenk

*MAKING LIFE EASY: A Simple Guide to a Divinely
Inspired Life,* by Christiane Northrup, M.D.

*OWN YOUR GLOW: A Soulful Guide to Luminous Living and
Crowning the Queen Within,* by Latham Thomas

All of the above are available at your local bookstore,
or may be ordered by contacting Hay House (see next page).

———

We hope you enjoyed this Hay House book. If you'd like to receive our online catalog featuring additional information on Hay House books and products, or if you'd like to find out more about the Hay Foundation, please contact:

Hay House, Inc., P.O. Box 5100, Carlsbad, CA 92018-5100
(760) 431-7695 or (800) 654-5126
(760) 431-6948 (fax) or (800) 650-5115 (fax)
www.hayhouse.com® • www.hayfoundation.org

———

Published in Australia by: Hay House Australia Pty. Ltd.,
18/36 Ralph St., Alexandria NSW 2015
Phone: 612-9669-4299 • *Fax:* 612-9669-4144
www.hayhouse.com.au

Published in the United Kingdom by: Hay House UK, Ltd.,
The Sixth Floor, Watson House, 54 Baker Street, London W1U 7BU
Phone: +44 (0)20 3927 7290 • *Fax:* +44 (0)20 3927 7291
www.hayhouse.co.uk

Published in India by: Hay House Publishers India,
Muskaan Complex, Plot No. 3, B-2, Vasant Kunj, New Delhi 110 070
Phone: 91-11-4176-1620 • *Fax:* 91-11-4176-1630
www.hayhouse.co.in

———

Access New Knowledge.
Anytime. Anywhere.

Learn and evolve at your own pace
with the world's leading experts.

www.hayhouseU.com

Listen. Learn. Transform.

Embrace vibrant, lasting health with unlimited Hay House audios!

Unlock endless wisdom, fresh perspectives, and life-changing tools from world-renowned authors and teachers—helping you live your happiest, healthiest life. With the *Hay House Unlimited* Audio app, you can learn and grow in a way that fits your lifestyle . . . and your daily schedule.

With your membership, you can:

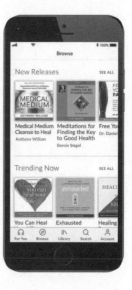

- Develop a healthier mind, body, and spirit through natural remedies, healthy foods, and powerful healing practices.

- Explore thousands of audiobooks, meditations, immersive learning programs, podcasts, and more.

- Access exclusive audios you won't find anywhere else.

- Experience completely unlimited listening. No credits. No limits. No kidding.

Try for FREE!

Visit **hayhouse.com/try-free** to start your free trial and get one step closer to living your best life.